Asperger Syndrome in Adults

Dr Ruth Searle began her career as a nurse and midwife and, although her love of nursing has remained constant, she went on to fulfil her dream of becoming a marine biologist. She completed her PhD on humpback whale behaviour and is continuing with field research that takes her around the world. Passionate about nature, wildlife and conservation, she writes about the subjects she loves, including marine biology and the humpback whale. Ruth confesses to being 'hooked' on studying: she recently completed a second degree in Earth sciences, cosmology and particle physics, and plans to study philosophy next. Her triumphs and struggles to find and live her own personal dreams provide the inspiration for much of her writing, including *The Thinking Person's Guide to Happiness*, *Coping with Compulsive Eating* and *Overcoming Shyness and Social Anxiety*, all published by Sheldon Press.

Overcoming Common Problems Series

Selected titles

A full list of titles is available from Sheldon Press,
36 Causton Street, London SW1P 4ST and on our website at
www.sheldonpress.co.uk

Asperger Syndrome in Adults
Dr Ruth Searle

The Assertiveness Handbook
Mary Hartley

Assertiveness: Step by step
Dr Windy Dryden and Daniel Constantinou

Backache: What you need to know
Dr David Delvin

Body Language: What you need to know
David Cohen

The Cancer Survivor's Handbook
Dr Terry Priestman

The Chronic Fatigue Healing Diet
Christine Craggs-Hinton

The Chronic Pain Diet Book
Neville Shone

Cider Vinegar
Margaret Hills

The Complete Carer's Guide
Bridget McCall

Confidence Works
Gladeana McMahon

Coping Successfully with Pain
Neville Shone

Coping Successfully with Period Problems
Mary-Claire Mason

Coping Successfully with Prostate Cancer
Dr Tom Smith

Coping Successfully with Psoriasis
Christine Craggs-Hinton

Coping Successfully with Ulcerative Colitis
Peter Cartwright

Coping Successfully with Varicose Veins
Christine Craggs-Hinton

Coping Successfully with Your Hiatus Hernia
Dr Tom Smith

Coping Successfully with Your Irritable Bowel
Rosemary Nicol

Coping When Your Child Has Cerebral Palsy
Jill Eckersley

Coping with Age-related Memory Loss
Dr Tom Smith

Coping with Birth Trauma and Postnatal Depression
Lucy Jolin

Coping with Bowel Cancer
Dr Tom Smith

Coping with Candida
Shirley Trickett

Coping with Chemotherapy
Dr Terry Priestman

Coping with Chronic Fatigue
Trudie Chalder

Coping with Coeliac Disease
Karen Brody

Coping with Compulsive Eating
Dr Ruth Searle

Coping with Diabetes in Childhood and Adolescence
Dr Philippa Kaye

Coping with Diverticulitis
Peter Cartwright

Coping with Eating Disorders and Body Image
Christine Craggs-Hinton

Coping with Epilepsy in Children and Young People
Susan Elliot-Wright

Coping with Family Stress
Dr Peter Cheevers

Coping with Gout
Christine Craggs-Hinton

Coping with Hay Fever
Christine Craggs-Hinton

Coping with Headaches and Migraine
Alison Frith

Coping with Hearing Loss
Christine Craggs-Hinton

Coping with Heartburn and Reflux
Dr Tom Smith

Coping with Kidney Disease
Dr Tom Smith

Coping with Life after Stroke
Dr Mareeni Raymond

Overcoming Common Problems Series

Overcoming Common Problems Series

Overcoming Common Problems

Asperger Syndrome in Adults
A guide to realizing your potential

DR RUTH SEARLE

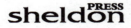
sheldon**PRESS**

First published in Great Britain in 2010

Sheldon Press
36 Causton Street
London SW1P 4ST
www.sheldonpress.co.uk

British Library Cataloguing-in-Publication Data
A catalogue record for this book is available from the British Library

ISBN 978–1–84709–069–0
1 3 5 7 9 10 8 6 4 2

Typeset by Fakenham Photosetting Ltd, Fakenham, Norfolk
Printed in Great Britain by Ashford Colour Press

Produced on paper from sustainable forests

Contents

Acknowledgements

My very grateful thanks to Fiona Marshall for her help and support, and to the editorial and production teams at Sheldon Press.

Introduction

Someone with Asperger syndrome thinks and perceives the world differently from the way the majority of people do. I describe it like this deliberately because, increasingly, there is a debate as to whether Asperger syndrome should be labelled as a disorder or simply as a different way to think and behave than is common or typical in the general population. It was only recently, in the mid 1940s, that these differences were 'labelled' as Asperger syndrome by a Viennese paediatrician, Hans Asperger.

Has it helped to give people a label and a diagnosis? This is a question that we will explore throughout the course of this book. Ultimately only you can decide whether being categorized as someone with Asperger syndrome is beneficial. There is a growing feeling, however, that, rather than believing you have something wrong with you, it is better to celebrate your differences, stand up and be proud of who you are.

Asperger syndrome, of course, manifests itself in a variety of ways, some mild and some more severe. This book is largely designed to help those of you whose condition is at the milder end of the spectrum. Those whose condition is more severe may find another book, *Living with Asperger Syndrome* by Dr Joan Gomez (also published by Sheldon Press), more helpful.

Even if your condition is relatively mild, however, there are difficulties in having Asperger syndrome in a world where most people think and behave in a typical way – in this book we'll call them neurotypical. But we mustn't forget that there are also great advantages and compensations in being atypical.

I am firmly with the growing wave of people – including numerous researchers, as well as people with Asperger syndrome who are rebelling against being labelled with a disorder or a disability – who believe that those with Asperger syndrome have a great deal to give to the world *just as they are*. If you have been diagnosed with Asperger syndrome, I want you to know that you have many of the special qualities and valuable characteristics that humankind has always needed throughout its history. You have qualities that are just as vital and important today as they have always been – labelled or not.

However, simply being in any minority is difficult. But knowledge brings the strength to cope, while awareness enables you to make your own decisions about the issues. In this book, therefore, we will first investigate and discuss Asperger syndrome in adults as a disorder: what it is, the symptoms, diagnosis and experience of having Asperger syndrome. Then we will explore the argument that the traits of Asperger syndrome can be seen as a variation of normal behaviour. Finally, we will discuss how you can overcome some of the difficulties associated with Asperger syndrome and get the most out of life, understand your relationships better and cope with your differences.

So let's now explore some of the aspects of Asperger syndrome – both as a disorder, requiring treatment in the form of counselling, therapy or even medical intervention, and as a simple difference to be celebrated and enjoyed.

1

What is Asperger syndrome?

Asperger syndrome is a form of autism and is classified as part of the autism spectrum of disorders, which includes high-functioning autism, and a broader class called 'pervasive developmental disorders' (PDDs) or 'pervasive developmental disorder – not otherwise specified' (PDD – NOS), both very mild forms of autism. It is characterized by difficulty in social interactions and communication, distinctive patterns of behaviour and intense, narrowly focused interests. People with Asperger syndrome may also use language atypically and may display clumsiness, although these are not required to be evident for a diagnosis to be made.

Asperger syndrome begins in infancy or childhood and is present throughout life to varying degrees. Some people who show Asperger-like traits in their social behaviour will not be diagnosed with Asperger syndrome. There is no 'cure' for Asperger syndrome, although behavioural therapy can help people with Asperger syndrome to cope with and improve their social interactions and communicate more effectively.

There is debate about the causes of Asperger syndrome, but it *may* be caused by genetic differences in brain structure, although brain imaging techniques such as functional magnetic resonance imaging (fMRI) scans have not proved conclusively that there is any pathology involved.

History of Asperger syndrome

Asperger syndrome is a relatively new condition to be added to the range of autism disorders. It was described by Hans Asperger in 1944 when he documented the social isolation and behaviour of children in his practice as a paediatrician at the University Children's Hospital in Vienna. These children were described as having difficulty with social integration, lacking non-verbal

1

communication skills and being unable to show empathy with others. They were also physically clumsy. He called the condition 'autistic psychopathy' (autism means 'self' and psychopathy means 'disease of the personality'). He called his patients 'little professors', due to their ability to talk so knowledgeably and in such detail on their favourite subjects. He believed many of the children he studied would go on to achieve extraordinary success in their adult lives. Indeed one of Asperger's patients, Elfriede Jelinek, was awarded a Nobel Prize for literature in 2004 for her writing as a novelist and feminist playwright.

Hans Asperger himself was described as distant and lonely as a child. He had difficulty making friends and displayed aspects of what he later identified as Asperger syndrome. Asperger set up a school for children with autistic psychopathy towards the end of the Second World War. However, the school was bombed and much of his early work was lost. His paper on Asperger syndrome was published in German and was not widely read at the time – he died in 1980, before his work was recognized.

Asperger syndrome is thought by some to be a form of high-functioning autism and the diverse work of both Asperger and Leo Kanner, an Austrian-American psychiatrist, formed the basis of the modern study of autism. Asperger syndrome was first popularized to the English-speaking medical community by Lorna Wing, an English psychiatrist, in 1981 through a series of case studies of children showing similar symptoms. Wing's own daughter was autistic and she became interested in researching autism spectrum disorders; she also founded the National Autistic Society (NAS) in the UK in 1962 (see Useful addresses at the end of the book for details of this and other organizations).

Later, in 1991, Uta Frith, a leading developmental psychologist, translated Hans Asperger's paper into English and by 1992, Asperger syndrome became a standard diagnosis. It was included in the World Health Organization's classification of diseases in 1992 and added to the American Psychiatric Association's manual of mental disorders in 1994.

Since then, hundreds of books and articles have been written on Asperger syndrome, and autism spectrum disorders and there are now many websites dedicated to the subject. Not surprisingly, the estimated prevalence of people with Asperger syndrome has increased dramatically due to this increased awareness among both professionals and the general public. The debate continues among clinicians, researchers and people with the condition as to whether it should be called a syndrome, a disorder, or indeed whether it should simply be left as a neurological difference.

Prevalence of Asperger syndrome

Because of variations in the criteria for diagnosing Asperger syndrome, there are widely differing estimates of its prevalence. Also, there is no register of people with autism or Asperger syndrome in the UK, so it is all the more difficult to estimate the prevalence of the condition.

Estimates of the prevalence of Asperger syndrome in children range, depending on the diagnostic criteria, between 0.3 per 10,000 and as many as 8.4 per 10,000 children (which equates to between 1 in 33,000 and 1 in 1,200 children). Some researchers suggest that as many as 1 in 70 schoolchildren are being diagnosed with some form of autism, somewhere along the autism spectrum. Clinical psychologist Tony Attwood believes that about 50 per cent of children with Asperger syndrome are currently being detected and diagnosed – the others are being missed by clinicians or managing to camouflage their difficulties and avoid detection.

The prevalence of Asperger syndrome in adults is notoriously difficult to estimate because many people with Asperger syndrome do not seek a diagnosis, or have developed sufficient skills to overcome their difficulties. However, from the figures that are available, there are an estimated 1 per 1,000 adults with Asperger syndrome, although some experts say it is as high as 1 in 300. According to the National Autistic Society, there are 588,000 people with autism, including Asperger syndrome, in the UK today, although this is likely to be an underestimate. It is found at least ten times more commonly in males than females, according to Professor Simon Baron-Cohen of the Autism Research Centre at Cambridge University.

The characteristics of Asperger syndrome

Let's discuss in more detail the characteristics of Asperger syndrome as a lifelong condition. The basic characteristics include impaired communication and social interactions, as well as repetitive behaviour and a preoccupation with a narrow subject area. People with Asperger syndrome tend to hold long-winded and one-sided conversations and can be pedantic in their communication with others. They are usually highly intelligent and have no problems with language development in childhood.

Social interactions

Someone with Asperger syndrome tends to lack empathy with other people. The ability to show empathy first requires an ability to *recognize* the emotional state of another person. This is an important social skill when communicating with neurotypical people because it is often the only way really to understand what is important to them and establish a cooperative and productive relationship. Although the actions and words used by most people are fundamentally driven by their emotional state, it is perhaps surprising that many people don't necessarily 'spell out' how they are feeling at the time. We therefore need to listen to tone of voice or observe body language such as eye contact, posture, gesture and facial expression. For people with Asperger syndrome it is not impossible to develop and maintain friendships; it can however be quite challenging. Those with Asperger syndrome establish romantic relationships with difficulty and may not display socially accepted behaviours. However they are not generally shy or withdrawn around others, which is a positive attribute.

From the perspective of a neurotypical person, someone with Asperger syndrome may appear awkward or clumsy in social situations and have difficulty responding to non-verbal signals. For example, people with Asperger syndrome may have difficulty recognizing the *reactions* of someone listening to one of their long-winded speeches, and this can lead to inappropriate behaviour. People with Asperger syndrome may be considered insensitive to others' feelings and even though they may have a theoretical understanding of human emotions, they have difficulty in applying this knowledge to real-life situations. A willingness to try to socialize in the generally accepted way can result in awkward social interactions such as forced eye contact and rigid behaviour. Contrary to common belief, people with Asperger syndrome do not necessarily prefer to be alone – they enjoy social contact, despite the difficulties it might bring.

Case history: Peter

Peter had an impressive talent for information technology and his strong knowledge of computer architecture and operating systems was an asset to his employer. Peter's approach to his work was very exacting and he would not tolerate errors or inconsistencies in his work activities. There was no room for ambiguity and everything he was involved in was categorized in one way or another. Unfortunately, Peter's exacting approach to IT was also applied when it came to social situations. His wife had invited her friend Julie to dinner one evening. Julie was wearing a new dress and asked Peter and his wife what they thought about it. Although his wife was complimentary, Peter was compelled to point out that Julie was too fat to wear the dress and that the seam had stretched in the area of her waistline. At one level, Peter was being honest and he considered that this exact and diagnostic response was exactly what Julie had requested. In reality, Peter had not recognized that Julie was looking for compliments and only wanted to hear about the positive aspects of the new dress in a way that would help her forget about her weight problem. The impact of Peter's behaviour was far-reaching and Julie did not feel confident to visit their house in future. This made Peter's wife unhappy and she missed seeing her friend Julie on a frequent basis.

Everyone has some limitations in their capacity for social contact. Some people enjoy socializing, are extroverts and can happily interact with others for hours on end, but others tire of socializing quite quickly and may be introverts at heart. This is all perfectly understandable. People with Asperger syndrome may have a limited capacity for socializing because they are only able to achieve success in social interactions by intellectualizing and thinking about how social interactions work – they find it difficult to understand this process intuitively as neurotypical people do. This can be exhausting for anything more than a fairly short period of time.

Obsessive interests

People with Asperger syndrome may collect huge amounts of information on their favourite topic and will often dominate social interactions and conversations with long monologues about their particular interest. Many people with Asperger syndrome tend to have narrowly focused and intense interests which can be limited and repetitive. They may pursue a narrow topic, delving into the minutest detail without necessarily having a good understanding of the broader subject.

> *Case history: Timothy*
> Timothy is 29 and his behaviour is typical of someone with Asperger syndrome. He has an impressive and highly detailed knowledge of the postal code system, yet it is significant that many of the people who know Timothy have a low tolerance of him because of his preoccupation with the topic of post codes. On a recent walk through his local park, Timothy sat next to June on the park bench. He started to list a number of post codes for the district of Bradford. His list began with BD1 1TG, BD1 3PZ, BD3 8DS, BD8 9BN and how these numbers corresponded to shops and places close to Bradford town centre. At no point did Timothy ask June about her interest in the topic of post codes or try to explore a point of common interest (perhaps a holiday town). He continued listing more and more post codes and covered some for the Leeds area including LS2 8DG, LS1 5ER and LS2 7RQ. At one point June tried to change the subject, but Timothy's lecture on post codes continued for 15 minutes. Although Julie did not want to tell him how bored she was feeling, her body language was obvious to passers-by – she was resting her chin on her hand and looking away from him. June did not want to appear rude or to abandon Timothy but her feeling of boredom became so intense that she simply had to do something to escape from the situation. So she pretended that she recognized a friend across the park and raced off towards the person she saw, leaving Timothy on his own.
>
> Timothy very much likes to be near other people and feels happier in company than on his own. Unfortunately, similar experiences to the one he had with June have happened many times in the past. He knows that somehow he gets stuck in a groove and can't seem to move out of it.

Movements

People with Asperger syndrome often display stereotypical and repetitive physical behaviours such as twisting or flapping hand movements and strange, sometimes complex movements of the body, which appear to be ritualistic and voluntary (rather than involuntary movements such as tics or spasms). They may have an unusual gait or posture.

There may be a delay during childhood in developing motor skills and dexterity such as riding a bicycle. People with Asperger syndrome may have poor coordination or balance and move awkwardly.

Case history: Colin
Colin is a 22-year-old man with Asperger syndrome and has always had a habit involving his hands. When he is talking to one of his friends he tends to intertwine his fingers so that his palms face upwards and his fingers point towards his face. As he talks, he flexes his fingers from side to side and keeps this up until he is alone or stops talking. As a boy, he used to get teased and bullied by other boys and they would push him over to see if he could unclasp his hands to break his fall. Colin has never wanted to stop his hand movement and does not always notice that he is doing it. There is of course no reason why he should stop; however, it appears to other people as something different and unusual, and there- fore gets noticed and even commented on.

Communication

People with Asperger syndrome tend to interpret speech liter- ally and are unable to comprehend double meanings, the use of metaphor and some types of humour. They may be unable to understand certain jokes, irony and teasing, for instance, although some individuals have a good grasp of humour, so this aspect of Asperger syndrome is not universal.

They tend to be pedantic and very formal in their speech, with oddities in certain aspects of speech such as intonation, pitch or volume. This can lead to idiosyncratic patterns of speech, which can be jerky, too quiet or too loud.

While people with Asperger syndrome often have a wide vocabu- lary, which develops at a young age, they may have difficulty in understanding figurative language or the meaning of some of the words they use in conversation.

Case history: Tom

Tom is 32 and lives with his mother in a rural area outside Blackpool. He has no brothers or sisters and his father left home when he was 12 years old. Unfortunately, Tom has never established many friendships and tends to spend most of his spare time with his mother at home and developing his collection of butterflies. Tom is competent in explaining himself and describing features of his collection. His voice and speech are consistent and smooth and always at the same pitch and volume. In the evening he will often sit with his mother and tell her about his hobby. Unfortunately, she has heard much of it before and the 'soft' tone of his voice sends her off to sleep. Tom has always admired some of the presenters on TV nature programmes. He wonders how they make the subject sound so interesting and why they get so many emails and enquiries from viewers. He asks himself, 'Is it something about their detailed knowledge of the subject?'

The neuropsychology of Asperger syndrome

Asperger traits in the general population

In 2006 Professor Simon Baron-Cohen ran an Autism-Spectrum Quotient test (AQ) on four groups of people: 58 adults with Asperger syndrome and 74 randomly selected controls, 840 students at Cambridge University and the 16 winners of the UK Mathematics Olympiad.[1] Each group was sent a questionnaire covering the autistic traits of social skill, attention switching, attention to detail, communication and imagination. The results showed that the majority of people with Asperger syndrome scored above 32 out of a maximum of 50 on the AQ. The interesting thing was that science and technology students at Cambridge University had a higher AQ score than students in the arts and humanities. Mathematicians scored the highest of all the non-Asperger groups, with around 20 out of 50, closely followed by engineers, computer scientists and physicists. Among the scientists, biologists and medics scored the lowest with around 14 out of 50.

This experiment showed that autistic traits are actually very common in the general population – it is the people with a large number of these traits that end up being diagnosed with Asperger syndrome.

An autism epidemic?

Over the past 10 to 15 years, around the world, there has been a dramatic rise in the number of cases of autism. This has led many people to believe that we have an autism epidemic. Such a sudden rise in the number of cases of a condition tends to indicate that an environmental factor, rather than a genetic factor, may be responsible, and many theories have been put forward to account for the rise in the number of cases of autism. These include suggestions that the combined measles, mumps and rubella (MMR) vaccine, mercury in vaccines (in the USA), food allergies, antibiotics and viral infections may be responsible – none of which have any solid scientific evidence to support them. A recent report by Professor Baron-Cohen in the USA has linked the rise in Asperger syndrome with the introduction of cable television and its influence on the development of young children. Research has shown that children with Asperger syndrome have unusual activity in parts of the brain that process visual information and these areas develop in early years.

On the other hand, Brent Taylor, a professor of Community Child Health at University College London, does not believe there has been any increase in the incidence of autism, and asserts that there is no autism epidemic. His beliefs are supported by many studies that have failed to find an increase in the prevalence of autism.

There are various possible explanations for the rise in the number of cases of autism. Diagnosis itself is highly subjective – there is no definitive test – and since 1980 the diagnostic criteria have been revised five times, broadening the definition of autism and including many at the less severe end of the spectrum, people who would previously never have been considered to have Asperger syndrome or pervasive developmental disorders. Tellingly, around three-quarters of all the more recent diagnoses of autism are for the milder types, specifically, Asperger syndrome and PDD – NOS. This could be due to several factors.

First, there has been a huge increase in public awareness of autism among both the public and health care workers and clinicians. Professor Taylor points out that 20 years ago there were maybe ten autism specialists in the UK – now there are over 2,000.

Second, there is less of a stigma in having autism, encouraging more parents and adults to seek a diagnosis. Also, there are more services and help available for people who are diagnosed with autism and this has encouraged doctors to include ambiguous or borderline cases in order to qualify for this help.

In 2001, Helen Heussler of Nottingham University and her team re-examined data from a 1970 survey of 13,135 British children. Originally, the survey found just five autistic children, but using modern diagnostic criteria, they found a further 56 children – a tenfold rise in numbers. Either the earlier study seriously underestimated the prevalence of autism, or the rise is due to a broadening of the diagnostic criteria. However, Lorna Wing, an autism researcher at the Institute of Psychiatry in London, believes that in the 1970s many people were diagnosed incorrectly, and the prevalence of autism was underestimated. She believes that our prisons and institutions are full of people with autism who have been wrongly diagnosed with conditions such as schizophrenia.

Ultimately, there is no clear evidence either to prove or disprove the existence of an autism epidemic, but there *is* plenty of evidence to suggest that there is no environmental problem that triggers autism, or that upbringing and parenting is in any way responsible for autism.

Famous people with Asperger syndrome

You are definitely not alone if you have Asperger syndrome. There are many famous people with Asperger syndrome, along with the half a million or so people in the UK who are not so well-known. There is no space to list them all, but the following is a small selection of well-known people with diagnosed Asperger syndrome:

Gary Numan, a British singer, songwriter and musician. He had several hits in the 1970s and 1980s and is widely known for his chart-topping hits in 1979, 'Cars' and 'Are Friends Electric?' In 2001, Gary gave an interview in which he said, 'Polite conversation has never been one of my strong points. Just recently I actually found out that I'd got a mild form of Asperger's syndrome which basically means I have trouble interacting with people. For years, I couldn't understand why people thought I was arrogant, but now it all makes more sense.'

Dawn Prince-Hughes, an anthropologist, primatologist and ethologist with a PhD from the University of Herisau in Switzerland. She has studied gorilla behaviour and is associated with the Jane Goodall Institute. She is the author of several books including *Songs of the Gorilla Nation*, in which she wrote about how she learned techniques to manage her Asperger syndrome, and escape social isolation, through her work observing and interacting with gorillas.

Peter Howson, a Scottish painter with work exhibited in many major collections, including the private collections of David Bowie, Mick Jagger and Madonna. He was the official artist in the Bosnian civil war in 1993, when he portrayed some of the atrocities that took place. His work has also appeared on album covers by Live, Jackie Leven and The Beautiful South.

Richard Borcherds, a British mathematician specializing in lattices, number theory, group theory and infinite-dimensional algebras. He has studied and worked at Cambridge University and has held a Royal Society Research Professorship there. He is currently Professor of Mathematics at the University of California, Berkeley. In 1998 he was awarded the Fields Medal, which is considered the highest honour a mathematician can receive.

Tim Page, a Californian writer, editor, producer and professor. He is also a music critic for the *Washington Post* and has won the Pulitzer Prize for his music criticism. He wrote the biography of American author Dawn Powell and in 2008, he joined the faculty of the University of Southern California. He publicized in the *New Yorker* that he had finally been diagnosed with Asperger syndrome, 'in a protracted effort to identify, and possibly alleviate my lifelong unease'.

Peter Tork, an American musician and actor, best known as a member of The Monkees. He appeared in a long-running TV show featuring the group, and after finishing with The Monkees started his own group called Release. In 2008, Peter became an advice columnist with an online advice and information column called Ask Peter Tork (<www.thedailypanic.com>).

Vernon Lomax Smith, a professor of economics at Chapman University, California. With a PhD from Harvard University, he shared the Nobel Memorial Prize in Economic Sciences with Daniel Kahneman in 2002. He has authored or co-authored over 200 articles and books on capital theory, finance, natural resource economics and experimental economics. In February 2005, he spoke publicly about his Asperger syndrome.

People speculated to have Asperger syndrome

Since Asperger syndrome has only been recognized since the 1940s, many cases prior to (and indeed since) this time would not have been diagnosed. There has been much speculation about whether the behaviour of certain famous people indicates that they had autism spectrum disorders. Fred Volkmar, a psychiatrist and autism expert at Yale Child Study Centre, says, 'There is a cottage industry of speculation as to who has Asperger syndrome.'

For example, some autism researchers have speculated that Wolfgang Amadeus Mozart had autism. Others speculated to have had Asperger syndrome include writers such as Hans Christian Anderson, Lewis Carroll, Arthur Conan Doyle, Herman Melville and George Orwell; musicians such as Ludwig van Beethoven and Bob Dylan; artists such as Vincent van Gogh, L. S. Lowry and Andy Warhol; philosophers such as Simone Weil; and leaders and politicians such as Thomas Jefferson and Keith Joseph. Even Charles Darwin, famous for his work on the theory of evolution, and Paul Dirac, a British mathematician awarded the Nobel Prize in Physics for his work on quantum mechanics, have been speculated to have had Asperger syndrome.

Albert Einstein was thought to have had Asperger syndrome and since his brain was preserved, we may know for sure when details of the physical features of the brain that are involved with the condition are discovered. Several authorities have suggested that Einstein had an Asperger-like personality, including Ioan James, Michael Fitzgerald and Tony Attwood. It has also been suggested that Isaac Newton had Asperger syndrome. Both scientists had intense scientific interests in specialized fields, to the extent that they would get so carried away they would forget to eat.

Einstein did not learn to speak until he was two or three years old and until the age of seven he tended to repeat sentences many times. As an adult, he was absent-minded and obsessed with his scientific work and he lacked a need for direct contact with other people. Despite this, he had a passion for social justice and social responsibility.

Newton was profoundly antisocial, spoke very little and was considered eccentric. He would speak to an empty room if no one attended his lectures!

Others disagree that either Einstein or Newton had Asperger syndrome, including Oliver Sacks and psychiatrist Glen Elliot of the University of California at San Francisco. Both men were geniuses, which is often associated with eccentric behaviour, intense passion for one's subject, social ineptitude, isolation and impatience with people who are less intellectual than oneself. However, this does not imply that they had Asperger syndrome.

In the next chapter, we turn our attention to the inner world of people with Asperger syndrome and explore in greater detail what it feels like to be someone with this condition.

2

What does it feel like to have Asperger syndrome?

In the last chapter we looked in general terms at some of the characteristics displayed by people with Asperger syndrome. Now we will explore in more detail the 'inner world' of people with Asperger syndrome and attempt to connect with their experiences and feelings. It is valuable to appreciate the perspective of those with Asperger syndrome and recognize the challenges that they face. Most of the difficulties described are more acute in autistic people and some of the examples refer to these extreme cases.

What are the problems associated with Asperger syndrome?

People with Asperger syndrome describe the following associated problems and feelings:

- loneliness;
- despair;
- feeling isolated;
- being misunderstood;
- not being wanted in a team or group;
- feeling uninterested in relating to others socially and not really caring about it;
- feeling alone, even in the company of others, or in a relationship with someone;
- experiencing a feeling of missing out on the social interactions that most people consider to be so important;
- feeling grief and loss at not being able to socialize or communicate in the way neurotypical people do;
- feeling socially lost;
- awakening to the realization of being egocentric;

- feeling disdain for the way neurotypical people make assumptions about the behaviour of someone with Asperger syndrome;
- exhaustion at trying to pretend to be 'normal';
- frustration at not being able to understand how others feel when they socialize;
- sadness and despair at knowing there is no cure;
- finding that the more connection there is with others, the greater the realization that the differences are profound;
- struggling to accept Asperger syndrome;
- frustration with professionals who are trying to help people with Asperger syndrome 'appear normal' – when all they want is to be accepted for who they are;
- resentment at having to learn how not to alienate other people;
- anxiety about being rejected by others;
- frustration at being told how they are supposed to feel if they were 'normal';
- sadness that they will never have the same perspective that neurotypical people have;
- anxiety about being accepted;
- anxiety about making a mistake;
- anxiety about looking 'stupid' in a social situation;
- feeling trapped with nowhere to go;
- being treated like a child;
- wanting to be respected as an individual;
- being discriminated against for having a disorder, or not being considered 'normal';
- frustration at the lack of support offered for people with Asperger syndrome.

Asperger syndrome in social situations

The majority of the problems associated with having Asperger syndrome are related to interactions with other people in social situations, and in intimate relationships. Since people with Asperger syndrome don't always see the *full picture*, relationships and social interactions can prove to be extremely difficult for all parties involved. Everyday things that most people take for granted, such as recognizing someone's face or reading someone's expression, can be difficult. Because people with Asperger syndrome focus

exclusively on the details of someone's face, they can have difficulty recognizing the overall expression, and this is why non-verbal
signals and body language are so hard for them to read. This does
become easier with time and experience. During a conversation,
someone with Asperger syndrome tends to remember the details
of the information being relayed but not the overall story. He may
have difficulty summarizing what is being said, and may contribute
too much irrelevant detail to a conversation.

When faced with a situation where there is a great deal of
activity and conversation, such as a crowded party, neurotypical
people are able to prioritize information and pick out the important
bits to concentrate on, usually the people, social interactions and
the conversation. However, in the same situation, somebody with
Asperger syndrome can easily be overwhelmed and will tend to pick
out irrelevant details, such as the pattern in the curtain material.

Some people with Asperger syndrome dislike being hugged or
kissed – not necessarily because they do not welcome affection, but
because they find being hugged physically uncomfortable.

Given that many people with Asperger syndrome are intelligent
and certainly aware of their difficulties, it is usually painful and
frustrating to be socially disconnected. Many have a strong desire
to be as social as they can be. At the same time though there is
often a feeling of aversion resulting from difficult past experiences,
coupled with a lack of understanding and an inability to feel a sense
of joining in the shared experiences of others.

> *Roger talks about his experience in socializing*
> 'I feel quite anxious when I'm with groups of people, especially
> if they are strangers. I think that my communication is OK, but
> I have been told that I sometimes lose track of conversations
> and jump from one subject to another, or start talking about
> my favourite interest without knowing, sometimes at great
> length. Many people have commented that I have problems
> in starting and ending conversations. Most have noticed this
> happens during phone calls. When people are trying to end the
> conversation, I don't realize or notice the hints they are making
> and carry on talking.
>
> 'On occasions, I can misinterpret a situation and get con-
> fused about what exactly was meant by a comment or a
> set of instructions. If the confusion happens with someone I

know then I feel happy to ask them to explain. However, with strangers, I lack confidence and I don't like asking because it highlights my problems with communication.'

What are the positive aspects associated with Asperger syndrome?

While there are many problems with having Asperger syndrome (and most adults with Asperger syndrome do not feel there are any benefits), it is not all negative – some positive aspects are reported. In her research, specialist counsellor Maxine Aston found that 40 per cent of respondents managed to find at least one advantage from having Asperger syndrome. These generally relate to abilities associated with work or special interests and the capacity for amazing concentration and focus. Here are some of the positive aspects:

- the ability to concentrate and focus;
- enhanced staying power for a particular project;
- the ability to see things through no matter how difficult or unpleasant they get;
- perfectionism, leading to outstanding results for any job undertaken;
- the ability to be patient;
- the ability to be objective and unbiased;
- the ability to be logical and pragmatic;
- the ability to take a logical, rather than an emotional approach to problem solving;
- modesty;
- honesty;
- loyalty to one's family;
- faithfulness to a partner;
- for many, high intelligence;
- for some, creative genius ...

Impact of the external environment

Many people with Asperger syndrome can suffer from sensory overload – a feeling of being overwhelmed by bright lights, noise or crowds. Situations such as shopping or parties can be highly uncomfortable and nerve-wracking. While we all find certain things irritating, people with Asperger syndrome tend to have unusual sensitivity to different sensory stimuli such as specific sounds, touch, light intensity, heat or cold, and the taste, smell and texture of different foods. They can also have an unusual sensitivity to pain and discomfort (either over-reacting or under-reacting).

People with Asperger syndrome have described a feeling of sensory overload, particularly in crowded, noisy situations. They may also distort or 'tune out' sensory stimuli and can be at various times both hyper- and hyposensitive to various sensory experiences.

Vision

Around one in five children with Asperger syndrome are sensitive to particular colours or bright light. Adults with Asperger syndrome have reported hypersensitivity to intense levels of light and sound and may show sensitivity to particular colours. They can also find visual stimuli confusing; many people with Asperger syndrome can never seem to find what they are looking for, even though it's right in front of them and plainly seen by other people.

Jane remembers her childhood and talks about her current difficulties with visual stimulation

'I liked the visual stimulation of watching automatic sliding doors, whereas another child might run and scream when he or she sees an automatic sliding door. A loud vacuum cleaner may cause fear in one autistic child and may be a pleasurable fixation to another child. When I look at moving sliding doors, I get the same pleasurable feeling that used to occur when I engaged in rocking or other stereotypical autistic behaviours.

'When I'm in a bright, noisy environment, like a crowded shop, the sensory stimulation seems to build up. It is almost like water filling up a bucket. It reaches the top and then spills all over the floor. That is what I feel like; I get swamped by the lights and noise and bustle and then my brain shuts down. Everything seems to come from the end of a long tunnel. I can't make out sounds, and sights barely make any sense. I end up barely aware of anything and I am usually only interested in getting away. I need somewhere quiet and familiar.

'The thoughts that I do remember passing through my head are so illogical and concern things that I would never even consider doing normally. That is one of my biggest fears – that I will act on one of those thoughts when overwhelmed. When I can't control it, or the stimulus is simply too much, I start breathing too fast, I perspire, I shake and get scared or irritable, I might indulge in stimulating activities like rubbing my leg. If I decide that more shopping is not necessary I may decide that what I've put in the basket so far isn't needed either.

'I sometimes zone out completely and any thinking is prolonged and difficult. My partner will help me refocus by using a method she and I have figured out, or she will simply remove me from the situation (get me to leave the shop). When engaged in an episode, I am barely able to maintain any verbal communication, and I have a hard time processing what others are saying to me. It isn't that I don't hear them ... I just can't decode it. I want to hide under a rack of clothes, or stay in the toilets, or go to a corner of the building. I find that I can't really see either. It's all a sort of big visual bright haze. Recovery can be a few minutes to the rest of the day in a familiar and relaxing environment.'

Sound

Several researchers have found that between 70 and 85 per cent of children with Asperger syndrome are sensitive to certain sounds. There appear to be three types of noise that people with Asperger syndrome describe as extremely unpleasant:

- sudden, sharp noises such as barking dogs, alarms, a telephone ringing, someone coughing, a plate smashing;
- high-pitched, continuous sounds such as the motors of vacuum cleaners, lawnmowers or hairdryers;
- complicated or confusing sounds such as a large social gathering or busy shopping centre.

Many bad behaviours are triggered by the anticipation of being subjected to a painful noise. Some autistic children will attempt to break the telephone because they are afraid it will ring. Common noises that cause discomfort in many autistic individuals are school bells, fire alarms, scoreboard buzzers in the gym, squealing microphone feedback and chairs scraping on the floor.

Jonathan talks about his sensitization to sounds
'My hearing is like having a sound amplifier set on maximum volume. My ears are like a microphone that picks up and amplifies sound. I have two choices: (1) turn my ears on and get deluged with sound or (2) shut my ears off. My mother told me that sometimes I acted like I was deaf, yet hearing tests indicated that my hearing was normal. I just can't modulate incoming auditory stimulation. I discovered that I could shut out painful sounds by engaging in rhythmic stereotypical autistic behaviour. Sometimes I 'tune out'. For example, I will be listening to a favourite song on the car radio and then later realize that I tuned out and missed half of the song. In college, I had to constantly take notes to prevent tuning out.

'I am unable to talk on the telephone in a noisy office or airport. If I try to screen out the background noise, I also screen out the voice on the telephone. When I was a child, I feared the ferry boat that took us to our summer holiday home. When the boat's horn blew, I threw myself on the floor and screamed. Autistic children and adults may fear dogs or babies because they are unpredictable, and can make a hurtful noise without warning. I liked the sound of flowing water and enjoyed pouring water back and forth between orange juice cans.'

Touch

Several researchers have found that over 50 per cent of people with Asperger syndrome are sensitive to specific types of touch. People with Asperger syndrome have reported unusual sensitivities to various tactile stimuli, for instance a hypersensitivity to the material of their clothing or the sensation of water on their body, or an aversion to normal social contact with people such as shaking hands. Others report pleasurable experiences from the same tactile stimuli. We all vary in our preferences for touch, but people with Asperger syndrome seem to have an unusually intense hyper- or hyposensitivity.

Temple Grandin describes her problems with touch sensitivity
Dr Temple Grandin is Assistant Professor of Animal Sciences at Colorado State University. She has an amazing understanding of animal behaviour and designs livestock handling facilities which reduce stress for animals. She has become a noted speaker on her personal experience of Asperger syndrome as well as her work with animals.

She is also the creator of the 'squeeze machine', a device developed to help people who are oversensitive to touch by increasing their tolerance to being touched and hugged. The machine compresses a person between two panels lined with foam pads, and helps to reduce stress, anxiety and nervousness.[2]

'I pulled away when people tried to hug me, because being touched sent an overwhelming tidal wave of stimulation through my body. I wanted to feel the comforting feeling of being held, but then when somebody held me, the effect on my nervous system was overwhelming.

'Small itches and scratches that most people ignored were torture. A scratchy petticoat was like sandpaper rubbing my skin raw. Hair washing was also awful. When mother scrubbed my hair, my scalp hurt. I also had problems with adapting to new types of clothes. It took several days for me to stop feeling a new type of clothing on my body, whereas a normal person adapts to the change from pants to a dress in five minutes. Many people with autism prefer soft cotton against the skin. I also liked long pants, because I disliked the feeling of my legs touching each other.

'Many autistic children will seek deep pressure. Many parents have told me that their children get under the sofa cushions or mattress. I craved deep pressure stimulation, but I pulled away and stiffened when my overweight aunt hugged me. In my two books, I describe a squeeze machine I constructed to satisfy my craving for the feeling of being held. The machine was designed so that I could control the amount and duration of the pressure. It was lined with foam rubber and applied pressure over a large area of my body.

'Gradually I was able to tolerate the machine holding me. The oversensitivity of my nervous system was slowly reduced. A stimulus that was once overwhelming and aversive had now become pleasurable. Using the machine enabled me to tolerate another person touching me. A partial explanation for the lack of empathy in autism may be due to an oversensitive nervous system that prevents an autistic child from receiving the comforting tactile stimulation that comes from being hugged. I learned how to pet our cat more gently after I had used the squeeze machine. I had to comfort myself before I could give comfort to the cat. It is important to desensitize an autistic child so that he/she can tolerate comforting touch. I have found that if I use my squeeze machine on a regular basis I have nicer images in my dreams. Experiencing the comforting feeling of being held makes nasty or mean thoughts go away.'

Smell and taste

According to the results of several pieces of research, over 50 per cent of those with Asperger syndrome are sensitive to smell and taste. Children with Asperger syndrome can be hypersensitive to smells that most other people don't even notice. This can also affect their sensitivity to the taste of food, leading to strange dietary preferences during childhood. Hypersensitivity to smell and taste may persist into adulthood, although children with extremely faddy diets may try a more varied diet as they grow older.

Janet talks about her sensitization to taste and smell
'I have what other people say are strange preferences for certain foods. I like the sharp taste of pickled onions and can't get enough of them. I can eat ten one after the other, and sometimes I like pickles combined with the soft taste of honey. I'll have custard on my potatoes and I hate the taste of chocolate – it's too bitter for me. Smells seem to be overpowering to me and I can't walk down the aisle in the supermarket where all the cleaning products are kept – it makes me sneeze and I feel very anxious. I ended up crying for an hour once after being bombarded with all the different smells – it was overpowering. Even walking through a crowd of people can be torture because I can smell all the different perfumes they are wearing and it's just too much. I have a fidget that helps me to keep calm. If I play with my pets or go on a swing that also seems to help.'

Body movement

People with Asperger syndrome often have an unusual lack of synchronization in their movements. This may exhibit itself as an odd gait or style of walking or running, difficulty with coordination or with maintaining posture, or involuntary tics.

The unusual patterns of movement and clumsy coordination are often picked up in childhood and may include impaired manual dexterity, balance, grasp and muscle tone. There may be symptoms of ataxia – difficulties with muscular coordination and unusual movements. Handwriting may also be a problem for many children and young adults with Asperger syndrome due to poor motor coordination. Many children with Asperger syndrome also have unusual facial expressions, with a flat, rigid expression that lacks the usual animated expression of emotions seen in most neurotypical people.

Between 20 and 60 per cent of children with Asperger syndrome develop involuntary tics which include twitches, nose twitching, grimacing, tongue protrusion, throat clearing, coughing, sucking sounds, hand-flapping, jerking and twisting. These involuntary movements generally reach a peak in early adolescence, but decrease over subsequent years. By about the age of 18, 40 per cent of children who earlier developed tics are free of them. Some tics can persist into adulthood as involuntary movements and sounds.

However, although many people with Asperger syndrome experience impaired movement and coordination skills, it does not necessarily affect sporting skills or the enjoyment of everyday life. With practice, many of their problems with movement and coordination can be overcome.

Kate talks about her walking

'I have always walked on the tip of my toes. It sort of helps me because it provides a greater sense of "feeling my body" and "knowing where it is in space". At times, I can feel some dizziness, and walking on my toes helps me to feel balanced and stops me feeling like I'm going to tip over.'

Communication and emotions

Given that communication of feelings is not commonplace for people with Asperger syndrome, it is understandable that many neurotypical people assume those with Asperger syndrome do not have any interest in or awareness of the feelings of others. This is not the case: people with Asperger syndrome can and do feel sympathy for others. They are certainly able to feel sadness, embarrassment, compassion and happiness for others. In fact, most people with Asperger syndrome have very intense feelings and emotions and are just as sensitive as the rest of the population. The only significant difference from neurotypical people is that for someone with Asperger syndrome the sharing of this information is not routine. However, people with Asperger syndrome will respond to questions about their emotions and can explain verbally what they are experiencing and feeling.

Like most people, those with Asperger syndrome have a range of trigger points for intense emotions. These triggers can result from a variety of situations. They may stem from an unexpected change in routine (e.g. if the swimming pool is late opening), or when something gets broken (e.g. if a string breaks when playing a guitar), or from an unexpected and personal remark made by someone.

Julian talks about how he has coped with emotions
'I was diagnosed with Asperger syndrome at the age of 44. In an emotional situation, I focus more on my own feelings and behaviour than those of the other person. I realize at that moment that I need some space and time (especially time) to think back on the other ways of interpreting what was actually going on. I know that during the "event" I really can't tell what is happening, the other person's intentions, etc. I try to get myself away from the situation as soon as possible. I try very hard not to get obsessed about it. I have someone I can trust to help me process the event. In a couple of days, sometimes longer, I feel more at ease, and I can then re-examine and re-frame what happened. However, some types of encounters are very traumatic and stay with me for a long time.

'In these situations, I often can't describe the emotion even though it can be strong and overwhelming. Afterwards, however, I make an effort to recognize what emotion that was (after having experienced that emotion again and matching it with the situation and circumstances in which I experienced it) and then finally I am able to label it.'

Empathy

Empathy is different from sympathy or pity; it is the capacity for you to know and understand what someone else is feeling, or the ability to put yourself in someone else's shoes. It involves understanding someone else's emotional states on a personal level – not simply recognizing an emotional state in general terms. For example, if you have a friend who is grieving over the death of a loved pet, empathy involves you imagining how that person feels and almost being able to feel it yourself – you are able to imagine being that person and experience the feeling yourself. If you do not feel empathy, then you might simply recognize that your friend feels grief, and have sympathy for her, but not be able to imagine how her grief might feel.

This ability to recognize the feelings of others, either those of another human or an animal, is called empathic recognition. It extends to recognizing other people's emotions through facial expressions and body language as well as verbal communication. People's tone of voice can give away how they are feeling – even over the phone – and an empathizer can sense the emotional atmosphere around others and pick up the general emotional state in a group of people. For example, if an empathizer walks in on a conversation at work between several people, he or she can immediately sense the emotional atmosphere – whether the group generally are distressed, anxious, excited or happy, for instance.

Two people can resonate with each other emotionally without necessarily having the capacity to feel empathy. It is essential for people to understand each other's emotions and their meanings but empathy goes further than that – it is about sharing the emotional state of another person and understanding it in relation to yourself.

People with autism, and usually those with Asperger syndrome, appear to have a reduced ability to demonstrate empathy with others. However, some researchers believe that this may be due to an inability to express empathy, not necessarily to feel it.

Communicating and socializing

Difficulties with communicating (verbally and non-verbally) and socializing are two key traits that are seen in those with Asperger syndrome. Communication difficulties are more apparent in family relationships, close friendships or intimate relationships and can cause misunderstandings and a great deal of frustration.

Many people with Asperger syndrome are less aware of people around them, and are less inclined to interact with others. They may be happy to be alone or to be engrossed in their own interests – even when there are other people present. During a social event, it is not unknown for someone with Asperger syndrome to ignore everyone else, wander off and do his or her own thing!

People with Asperger syndrome have little insight into how

other people think and feel and have difficulty imagining how their behaviour is perceived by others. This can result in inappropriate social behaviour, such as faux pas, and may result in them appearing odd to others. Communication is often strained or difficult and littered with misunderstandings, something which can be infuriating for all concerned. Socializing can be very unpredictable – a cause of much anxiety for someone with Asperger syndrome.

The extent to which communicating and socializing is problematic will vary among individuals with Asperger syndrome. Some people have more problems in certain areas than others and there are many varied factors which contribute to the overall picture, such as age, life experience, upbringing, intelligence and motivation. Some people are more able than others and so the following issues may or may not be problematic.

Indifference

People with Asperger syndrome tend to hate small talk and polite social chitchat because they cannot understand the need for it and have no desire to show interest in another person, when they have nothing in common with that person or are unlikely to need that person for anything in the future. Because those with Asperger syndrome are unable to comprehend other people's point of view or feelings, they cannot see the point in trying to make others feel welcome or engage in social trivia.

If they do not like somebody, people with Asperger syndrome find it hard, if not impossible, to hide the fact, unless they are obliged to interact with a person because he is superior at work – a boss, for instance – or is in some way relevant to their lives. However, if they see no point in interacting with a particular person, they may ignore that person, show their annoyance or simply walk away from him. Neurotypical people are more tolerant because they instinctively understand other people's feelings and perspectives and recognize accepted social conventions.

Maxine Aston conducted research which showed that just 20 per cent of men with Asperger syndrome expressed the desire to be liked and accepted by others. When they become aware of their own social failures, people with Asperger syndrome can become depressed and feel very isolated. Most, however, show indifference to whether or not they are liked and accepted and are not particularly motivated to improve their interactions with other people. They appear to be unaware of the consequences of their behaviour and this can cause a great deal of misery, frustration and embarrassment for their partners and family.

Selective hearing

Someone with Asperger syndrome has difficulty coordinating several different trains of thought – something that comes easily to most people. This can result in an apparently selective memory, where a person with Asperger syndrome only seems to remember bits of what he is being told. He can also take things completely out of context or fail to understand the point of what is being said. He may ask you about something you have just said, as if he did not hear it. As a result of tuning out and only hearing parts of a conversation, someone with Asperger syndrome may interpret almost everything that is being said as a criticism.

Misinterpretation

People with Asperger syndrome tend to interpret things literally and may not understand certain jokes, particularly sarcasm. This can create some rather bizarre conversations.

People also tend to exaggerate during conversations, such as saying that the queue for the bus was *miles* long, when it was in fact just a few feet long, or that it took *for ever* to get across town, when it actually took half an hour. Neurotypical people understand and accept these sorts of exaggerations in conversations, and realize that they are not to be taken literally. However, someone with Asperger syndrome does take them literally and will not readily understand these types of exaggerations.

Faux pas

People with Asperger syndrome tend to be very honest, but they have difficulty being tactful because they cannot imagine how someone else would feel. Because of this they can inadvertently cause offence with their remarks. In social situations, this is seen as rude and bad mannered and can cause embarrassment for people on the receiving end of such comments, as well as for partners or

friends of the person who is making them. It can also lead to appre-
hension about social events in the future, and anxiety about saying
the wrong thing.

Sex differences

Maxine Aston's research showed that women with Asperger syndrome tend to prefer, and get along better with, male friends than
other women. This could be because men make fewer emotional
demands on them. Men with Asperger syndrome often get on
better with women than with other men. This could be because
women tend to be more tolerant of a lack of social confidence and
make better listeners.

Due to lack of confidence, or just because they find someone
who is prepared to listen, people with Asperger syndrome can
become fixated on a particular person during a social event. This
can be misconstrued, particularly if the person is of the opposite
sex; it can be interpreted as being inappropriate, especially by that
person's partner! They also have difficulty reading body language
and may stand too close to other people or fail to read non-verbal
signals to back off. This can lead to awkwardness or anxiety for the
other person.

Sense of humour

It has been said that people with Asperger syndrome do not understand humour. However, many researchers, as well as others who
are close to someone with Asperger syndrome, dispute this. People
with Asperger syndrome have difficulty with certain types of
humour, such as sarcasm or double meanings, but they do have a
well-developed sense of humour.

Their sense of humour may be rather immature in its nature and
jokes can be repetitive – someone with Asperger syndrome may tell
the same joke over and over or take a practical joke to extremes.
Jokes can also become personal, embarrassing or offensive at times,
if they are aimed at someone in particular or are inappropriate to
the situation.

Thinking and memory

People with Asperger syndrome prefer to have strict routines and often work in occupations such as science, art, the law, accountancy, copyediting and other occupations that require careful attention to detail. Important areas for self-development are typically around planning, multitasking and dealing with abstract concepts. Although people with Asperger syndrome are very capable in working with details, they struggle to process these details into a coherent and wider picture and construct a working model for a broad area.

> *Simon talks about his visual thinking*
> 'When I think, it is mainly using "pictures" and I find it hard to think with words. In my mind I can play short movies almost at will. Until I became an adult I didn't even realize that many other people don't actually think in this way. The other day, I asked one of my friends to use their memory to picture a dog. If I think of a dog in my mind I see lots of movie clips with the dog doing different activities. I can even change the colour of the dog's fur or make the dog run backwards.'

Many people with Asperger syndrome think visually and will apply this to everything they do. In the working environment this can have a number of advantages, especially in fields like computer science or engineering design.

Working memory and recall

People with Asperger syndrome have difficulty switching their attention to a new topic when they are preoccupied with a particular train of thought – they have difficulty using their working memory. They need to complete one thought process before they can begin another. This can be seen as an inability to mentally 'multitask' or to keep track of more than one thing at once. People with Asperger syndrome sometimes monopolize a conversation and, as a consequence, hate to be interrupted when they are speaking.

Planning and time management

Problems with organization and planning can lead to poor time management and people with Asperger syndrome can appear to be disorganized. They may have difficulty judging time accurately or estimating how long it will take to finish a task, complete a journey, and so on. They tend to focus on current events and are less likely to talk about or plan events in the future. Indeed, they may have difficulty planning and preparing for the future. Because of their limited self-awareness, they also have difficulty projecting forward into the future lessons learned in the past – in other words, they have limited foresight (as well as limited hindsight). People with Asperger syndrome can have difficulty in adapting their day to fit in with a change. They tend to follow routines which become repetitive and obsessive. Many people with Asperger syndrome improve their organizational ability as they get older, but others constantly struggle with poor organization, planning and time management.

Susan talks about her memory

'Repeating things from movies and shows is always fun for autistic people. We tend to do that because it is an "order" thing; we know what is going to happen and when. Autistic people can often memorize any line for you and act it out with perfect voice imitation, but when it comes to tying your shoes or remembering to take a pill, etc. it seems that we can't remember how to do those things.'

3

Asperger syndrome: disorder or difference?

One of the big questions occupying researchers, individuals and groups involved with Asperger syndrome is whether it is a disorder or a difference. Is Asperger syndrome a disorder requiring help and treatment, or is it simply a difference in brain structure and behaviour which is atypical but still normal and not requiring treatment? And if it is a difference rather than a disorder, should we therefore help people with 'atypical' personalities to cope and try to fit in more with the majority of 'typical' people, or should we concentrate on helping 'typical' people to respect and interact effectively with 'atypical' people?

Neurodiversity

Neurodiversity is a term used to refer to differences in neurological development among normal human beings. It encompasses the vast majority of people with a typical (neurotypical) brain structure and its associated behaviour, as well as those with atypical brain structure and behaviour, including people with Asperger-like personalities and other related 'conditions' among the autism spectrum of 'disorders'.

The term neurodiversity was first used in 1998 in an article by Harvey Blume in the *New York Times*. It has since gained popularity among the online community of people with Asperger syndrome who are against a 'cure' and want to be accepted for who they are, along with their differences when compared to the so-called neurotypical (or NT, as they have become known) majority. The terms neurodiversity and neurotypical are also now used by the scientific community.

Scientists are beginning to find all sorts of distinct brain patterns that link to behaviour, enabling them to describe more and more

31

conditions and syndromes. Who knows how many more such syndromes or disorders will be discovered in the future? However, as neurologist Dr Antonio Damasio at the University of Iowa Medical Centre has said, only society can decide whether to accept these differences as disorders or to accommodate them as variations of normal. Where do we draw the line between what is normal and a condition that has to be labelled as something different?

As Damasio explained in the *New York Times* in 2004:

> What all of our efforts in neuroscience are demonstrating is that you have many peculiar ways of arranging a human brain and there are all sorts of varieties of creative, successful human beings ... for a while it is going to be a rather relentless process as there are more and more discoveries of people that have something that could be called a defect and yet have immense talents in one way or another.

Over the last two decades, there has been a general shift in awareness about brain function and the broad concept of intelligence. This is being driven partly by the theories of Howard Gardner, a Harvard education professor. Gardner believes that children who don't necessarily excel in the manipulation of words and numbers – so-called traditional intelligence – may do extremely well in other areas, including spatial reasoning.

The American Psychiatric Association has attempted to reduce the number of diagnoses of psychological disorders by imposing new criteria, such as a requirement that an individual must suffer from a defined impairment to qualify as having one of the 220 such disorders listed in its Diagnostic Statistical Manual. However, the definition of 'impairment' for each disorder is vague and not widely accepted. Many clinicians consider the diagnostic criteria too rigid to apply to individual cases and many experts argue that numerous new disorders and syndromes should be defined as differences and traits rather than medical diagnoses.

Others argue that a diagnosis may help people understand themselves and their behaviour and encourage others to be more tolerant of behavioural differences. Family members, for example, may make allowances for someone with a diagnosed disorder. (It should be noted, however, that many who advocate greater tolerance warn that it should not be used as an excuse for individuals to behave badly. Many individuals with mild symptoms have ample awareness of their own behaviour and are perfectly capable of adapting and compromising in order to get along with others. In this respect they are no different from anyone else – we all have to work at social relationships!)

In fact, there is a growing group of people with Asperger syndrome who consider themselves to be simply neurologically atypical and who humorously mock neurotypical individuals. An Internet site, the Institute for the Study of the Neurologically Typical (<www.isnt.autistics.org>), states that 'Neurotypical individuals find it difficult to be alone' and 'are often intolerant of seemingly minor differences in others'. It goes on to say that, 'tragically, as many as 9,625 out of every 10,000 individuals may be neurologically typical'.

This indicates the degree of indignation that some people feel at being labelled with a disorder or syndrome, and shows that there is a need to address these issues. It also shows that people with Asperger-like symptoms can, contrary to common belief, understand and enjoy humour!

Professor Simon Baron-Cohen has described his theory that, since the male brain is better at systemizing, while the female brain is better at empathizing, autism is nothing more than an extreme of the normal male brain. We will discuss this and other issues in more detail in the next chapter.

Disorder or difference? The arguments

For all the arguments that support the diagnosis of Asperger syndrome as a disorder, then, there are equally strong arguments that support the idea that it is an expression of neurodiversity.

Proponents of Asperger syndrome as a disorder claim that individuals with Asperger syndrome have reduced ability in certain cognitive areas such as theory of mind and executive functioning, and that they suffer developmental delays in communication and social understanding.

On the other hand, while these limitations may well cause problems for individuals and those close to them, there are compensations. Many people with Asperger syndrome have very genuine personalities, are honest and straight talking – they don't feel the need to tell white lies, they say what they think. You know where you stand with someone like this, and it makes for more honest relationships.

Perhaps the problem lies with neurotypical people and their lack of understanding of the differences. This unawareness can cause anxiety, stress and confusion, but does that necessarily mean that people with Asperger syndrome are impaired or deficient?

For relationships to work, especially when one partner has Asperger syndrome, a new perspective and a broader understanding and acceptance of the differences in human behaviour are required – but with the will to succeed, it can be done. We should remember that an individual with Asperger syndrome finds neurotypical behaviour equally baffling – which one is 'normal', and why can't society accept that differences don't necessarily indicate disorder? Why should someone who, for example, chooses to spend his time building computer systems be seen as doing something less valuable than someone who spends his time socializing?

We will come back to the arguments for and against the diagnosis of Asperger syndrome as a disorder during the course of the book, but in the meantime, here is a brief summary.

The arguments for Asperger syndrome as a 'disorder'

Theory of mind and executive functioning

Theory of mind is our ability to understand mental states and imagine other people's thoughts and feelings. It enables us to understand our own intentions, beliefs, feelings and desires, and imagine how the intentions, beliefs, feelings and desires of other people drive their behaviour. It is through theory of mind that we can predict and anticipate how other people might behave, an ability which begins in early childhood. After about the age of five, children are generally able to understand the behaviour and feelings of other people, and are capable of picking up social cues and responding appropriately.

People with Asperger syndrome have a limited theory of mind, which leads to a difficulty in anticipating and predicting other people's feelings and behaviour. They also have difficulty associating their own behaviour with the feelings of others. A limited theory of mind is fundamental to the difficulties in social interaction and communication seen in Asperger syndrome, many of which I described in the previous chapter.

Executive functioning is an aspect of the brain's operation that determines our conscious control of thoughts and behaviour. It is not involved with involuntary or routine functions such as breathing, eating and sleeping, but is a higher function that allows us to make decisions, plan ahead, organize and control our behaviour. Children develop executive functioning as they grow into adulthood, but those with Asperger syndrome will experience problems in areas of their thinking that involve planning, decision-making or complex organization. Executive functioning also includes working memory, inhibition and impulse control, self-reflection and self-monitoring, time management and prioritizing, as well as implementing new strategies and understanding abstract concepts.

Display of empathy

People with Asperger syndrome who are less socially focused, tend not to display empathy with other people.[3] When there are discrepancies in the level of empathy between people, it can cause considerable difficulties when one person does not *appear* to consider other people's perspective, thoughts and feelings.

A certain level of empathy is required for relationships to work, and when someone's feelings and opinions are frequently coldly disregarded, the relationship can become very difficult. This is one of the main arguments for retaining the term 'disorder' in relation to Asperger syndrome. We will discuss relationships in greater detail later in the book.

Accessing help

Another of the main arguments for continuing to regard Asperger syndrome as a disorder is that a recognized medical disability can qualify for specialist treatment, support and financial aid. This is especially important for the families of children with Asperger syndrome. Without a diagnosis, this sort of help is not available.

In adults, diagnosis and recognition of Asperger syndrome as a disorder can help individuals, partners, families, friends and colleagues understand the behaviour of the person concerned and address the relationship problems he or she may be having.

The arguments for Asperger syndrome as a 'difference'

Interpretation of behaviour

Professor Baron-Cohen describes 12 behavioural features of Asperger syndrome (particularly in children), based on diagnostic criteria that do not imply a disability:

1 more time spent with physical objects and systems than people;
2 communicates less than others;
3 tends to follow own desires and beliefs and is not easily influenced by others' desires and beliefs;
4 shows little interest in what the social group is doing or being part of it;
5 strong personal interests;
6 accurate perception of information;
7 good observation and recall;
8 different view of what is relevant and important in a situation;
9 fascination with patterns in shapes, dates or timetables, words and numbers (such as car number plates), lists;
10 fascination with systems, from simple systems such as plumbing or electrical systems to abstract systems such as mathematics;
11 strong desire to collect objects or information;
12 preference for experiences that can be controlled rather than anything unpredictable.

Several of these features can be seen as positive assets. Many neurotypical people are unable to think and form opinions for themselves and end up following the opinions of the masses, while great discoveries in science as well as changes in society are made and initiated by people with the courage and vision to think for themselves and form their own unique opinions. Another feature is good observation and recall – a quality many of us wish we could improve. There are many more features of Asperger syndrome that could be interpreted differently with a change of perspective.

Empathy for others

Although the *external* behaviour of people with Asperger syndrome can lack the communication of empathy, there is plenty of evidence to confirm that the associated feelings are felt and experienced *internally*. When we consider this similarity, it is not reasonable then to think of Asperger syndrome as a disorder.

Tony talks about his feelings of empathy

'When I began to understand my Asperger condition, I realized how different I was from many people. Having said that, I do not feel that I should change to become like a neurotypical person. I do feel emotions quite intensely; maybe my way of experiencing feelings is different from other people's, it's hard to prove that. I find it extremely difficult to express and talk to someone about my emotions in the same way that neurotypical people do. However, I do think I show love and emotion in a physical way. Alternatively, I like to shut myself away and write things down. My wife is now used to me sending her emails about how I feel.

'Much of my life has been about understanding who I am. It is sad that I have wasted so much time trying to be someone that I am not. Now I am older, I think I have learnt to accept myself for who I am. It's so unfair that others still judge me based on their own experiences. I think empathy is a very personal thing that can take a variety of forms, and I believe that neurotypical people should try to be a bit broader minded about this and not expect everyone to fit into a rigid structure.'

Temple Grandin talks about love

Dr Temple Grandin, Assistant Professor of Animal Sciences at Colorado State University, talks about how she experiences the emotion of love:[4]

'My brain scan shows that some emotional circuits between the frontal cortex and the amygdala just aren't hooked up – circuits that affect my emotions are tied to my ability to feel love. I experience the emotion of love, but it's not the same way that most neurotypical people do. Does this mean my love is less valuable than how other people feel?

'People need to remember that we are individuals and as diverse and different on the autism spectrum as those that are not. Society needs to stop expecting us to be something we are not, as true happiness never comes from feeling like a performing monkey! I can't be what I am not and I feel my biggest problem is other people's misconceptions on how I should be and the way they stereotype us into a generalization that is usually wrong for us. I may look like others, but I see, feel and express myself differently – that should be OK. Growing up, there were times when I felt 100 per cent misunderstood, so I tried even harder to please. Being continually expected to do things in a way which was strange to me, I grew up lacking confidence in myself. So for me now, I feel a fear of rejection and of expressing emotion in my own way, knowing it will be misunderstood. The logical side of me makes me feel that your way does not make sense and the perfectionist in me wants to get it right. It's like a barrier between me and those not on the autism spectrum. Another ASD person is no barrier and I connect with the person like a lost friend.'

Frustration with the neurotypical world

The idea that they have a disorder leads to frustration among many people with Asperger syndrome. These people do not feel they have a problem. Instead, they believe, the ways they give and receive, communicate and connect are clearly misunderstood by neurotypical people. Many feel and sense more about neurotypical people than is appreciated. Other people's moods can have a huge impact on those with Asperger syndrome and they can feel the need to escape and remove themselves from certain situations. They often feel that they have to do all the work in order to overcome the differences. This continual effort leads to a great deal of frustration about the 'neurotypical world', which can be quite draining, and it is healthy to be able to vent this frustration with like-minded people. Below are some extracts from various websites where people with Asperger syndrome speak out and 'turn the tables' on the 'neurotypical world'.

A comment on empathy from the Asperger's Parallel Planet forum:

> To me empathy is nothing more than a particular cluster of neurons firing in response to other neurons (probably the mirror neurons) in order that our species is able to perform certain tasks that are vital to group bonding.

And a comment on awareness, also from Asperger's Parallel Planet:

> I guess we are a difference within a difference and often from birth we grow up not being understood or allowed to be ourselves – wouldn't you be confused? Maybe it should be more about awareness, with those not on the autism spectrum showing more understanding and allowing us our differences.

The Institute for the Study of the Neurologically Typical website provides some insight from the autistic community and represents their views of the neurotypical population. One perspective describes neurotypical people as suffering from a neurobiological disorder characterized by preoccupation with social concerns, delusions of superiority and obsession with conformity. The website then goes on to explain that the diagnosis is confirmed when at least two of the following criteria are met:

A. Egocentrism (at least one of the following)
   (1) Egocentric perspective (e.g. fails to realize that others may have a different perspective, needs, nature, or experiences from his- or herself)
   (2) Egomania (e.g. acts or talks as though superior or more important than peers or others)
   (3) Selfishness (either or both of the following)
      (a) Marked greed or covetousness
      (b) Domineering or 'bossy' attitude
B. Lack of Originality (at least one of the following):
   (1) Rigidly follows traditions or social rituals
   (2) Is often 'faddish,' follow the latest fads, fashions, or 'crazes' invented or set by others
   (3) Often demonstrates a 'herd mentality' (e.g. thoughtlessly follows a social reference group or a local group of friends, often gives into 'peer pressure')
C. Lack of Sympathy (one or both of the following):
   (1) Cruel or callous towards the feeling of others (e.g. engages in teasing or ridiculing others, plays potentially harmful 'practical jokes' on unsuspecting victims who are unlikely to be amused)
   (2) Often manipulative (e.g. uses others as tools towards own goals, treats others as objects which may be acquired for own satisfaction, uses dishonesty as convenient way to achieve social goals).

These comments illustrate how strongly some people with Asperger syndrome feel about the way they are perceived and their need to redress the balance.

Humans are widely regarded as social animals, and a lack of sociability or communication is seen as a disability. However, this does not necessarily stand up to closer scrutiny. Everyone has different interests in life – this is completely normal! Some people love science, mathematics or technology, for example, and don't spend a great deal of time thinking about the intricacies of the social world. Others love psychology and thinking about human relationships, but spend very little time – if any – thinking about the scientific aspects of the world around them. It seems unfair, therefore, to label one person as disabled, when that person simply has different interests and abilities. Just as someone with Asperger syndrome has difficulty coping with the social world, a social psychologist would be equally impaired in the world of mathematics!

Society at large remains split about whether we should treat the condition and seek a cure for autism, or whether autism in its many forms should be accepted as a simple diversity in the way our brains process information. Many parents and people who are adversely affected by the more severe forms of autism disagree that it is simply a difference and call for more research and treatment. Severe autism can be extremely disabling and difficult for families to cope with.

However, many of the arguments for and against Asperger syndrome as a disorder are simply a matter of perception – a paradigm that can be shifted by an open mind.

4

Asperger syndrome as difference: changing perspectives

Now we've looked at the question of whether Asperger syndrome is a disorder or a difference, let's consider in more detail the evidence for regarding it simply as a difference between people with certain neurophysiological traits and neurotypical people. We'll also look at some of the issues that arise if we regard it as a difference. To save lengthy explanations every time I refer to people with Asperger syndrome or who exhibit Asperger-like traits, I will continue in this chapter to use the term 'people with Asperger syndrome' (or similar) when differentiating between people with those traits in their personality and neurotypical people. I'm trying in this way to accommodate both people who feel they have a disorder and those who feel they simply have a different type of personality.

Social and cultural aspects of Asperger syndrome

The Internet

The Internet has allowed all of us to communicate more readily with other people around the world. It has also allowed people with Asperger syndrome to contact and connect with others in the same situation. It has opened up many new opportunities to form relationships and join communities of people affected by Asperger syndrome.

Because communication and social interaction are difficult for people with Asperger syndrome, many people find it easier to communicate online than in person – it is easier to avoid non-verbal communication and the complexities of social contact via the Internet. It also filters out the sensory overload that so many people experience in crowds and social situations. The downside of all this is, of course, the lack of real human contact and the opportunity

41

to improve social skills through personal interactions. Also, because so much information (and misinformation) is available via the Internet, people can wrongly diagnose themselves. Nevertheless, thanks to this easy Internet contact, a whole new culture of language, discussion boards, chat rooms and social events has sprung up within the autism community.

Websites like Wrong Planet (see Useful addresses at the back of the book) have changed people's perceptions of Asperger syndrome, and provided support for the growing band of people campaigning for it to be seen not as a disorder, but simply a difference in the way our brains are wired – what we described in the previous chapter as neurodiversity. Wrong Planet is a great source of help, advice and camaraderie for people with Asperger syndrome, as well as a place for them to share frustrations. The content is wide ranging, including features such as limerick competitions. Here is an example:

> *Aspies are not all the same*
> *We vary from wild to tame*
> *And not all are wishin'*
> *To end the condition –*
> *But couldn't we PLEASE change the name?*

The Wrong Planet website is also an excellent source of advice on topics in response to 'Dear Aspie' questions; similar topics are covered later in this book, in the chapter on social relationships.

Campaign groups

Because so many people are beginning to see conditions along the autism spectrum as complex syndromes rather than diseases requiring treatment, there are now a number of campaigns promoting tolerance for neurodiversity. Movements such as Autistic Pride and Autistic Rights have been set up with the aim of encouraging society to accept and understand people with autism.

Autistic Pride Day, held on 18 June each year, is a celebration of the neurodiversity of people on the autism spectrum. Autistic pride is pride in autism. It is about shifting views of autism so that it is seen as 'difference' rather than 'disease'. Autistic pride emphasizes the innate potential in all human expressions and celebrates the diversity that various neurological types express. Autistic pride asserts that autistic people are not sick; rather, they have a unique set of characteristics that provide them with many rewards and challenges, not unlike their non-autistic peers. Researchers and people with high-functioning autism have contributed to a shift in attitudes away from the notion that autism is a deviation from the norm that must be treated or cured, and towards the view that it is a difference rather than a disability.

The London Autistic Rights Movement (London-ARM) is a civil rights organization representing the interests of autistic people to wider society. The aims of the group include campaigning for the civic and human rights of people on the autistic spectrum, the promotion of a positive autistic identity and the opposition of negative stereotypes.

Eccentricity

People who are considered eccentric usually display behaviour that is a bit unusual or odd – but certainly not maladaptive. Eccentricity is certainly not considered a disability. In fact, it is often perceived as an endearing quality. People with Asperger syndrome have their own uniquely eccentric characteristics, and there is no reason why these too cannot be accepted as a simple variation of 'normal'. Eccentricity is associated with creativity, originality and intelligence, and often associated with genius. As we saw in Chapter 1, Albert Einstein, a renowned eccentric, also showed many of the traits of Asperger syndrome.

People who are eccentric are considered original and not afraid to be different. They refuse to conform to society's norms and conventions and are happy to express their uniqueness and individualism – they are totally unconcerned by other people's opinions of them. Many people even deliberately develop eccentric behaviour or other unusual traits in order to differentiate themselves from the masses in the general population.

According to neuropsychologist David Weeks, there are several characteristics that may be considered eccentric in neurotypical people, including:

- a nonconforming attitude;
- creativity;

- intense curiosity;
- idealism;
- a happy obsession with a hobby or hobbies;
- a childhood realization that they are different from others;
- high intelligence;
- being outspoken and opinionated;
- lack of competitiveness;
- lack of interest in the opinions of others;
- happy to be alone – lack of interest in social or romantic relationships;
- unusual habits;
- a mischievous sense of humour;
- odd appearance and behaviour;
- beliefs and opinions that are not consistent with cultural norms;
- unusual speech, such as overly formal, pedantic speech.

When you read this list, you will see that many of the characteristics included are shared with people with Asperger syndrome. Yet eccentricity is not considered to be a disorder or condition needing treatment – it is considered a positive and charming characteristic. We admire and enjoy people who are eccentric. Perhaps Asperger syndrome should also be considered a form of eccentricity, rather than a disorder.

Eccentricity is a form of rebellion against social convention and authority, something the majority of us admire in those able to achieve it. Eccentric people assert their independence and their right to pursue their own interests without interference from governments, people in authority, or anyone else for that matter. It is a rebellion against the 'nanny state' and an antidote to the stresses of modern life.

British eccentricity

Whole countries have their own unique eccentricities and people around the world comment on the eccentricity of British people as a group, with our particular British characteristics, our mannerisms, habits, speech and cultural idiosyncrasies.

Eccentricity has been part of British culture for a very long time, as chronicled by the poet Edith Sitwell, herself the epitome of a twentieth-century eccentric. In her book, *English Eccentrics*, she gave some wonderful examples of eccentric English characters, many of them among the aristocracy – although eccentricity is by no means confined to the upper classes, and eccentrics are to be found in all walks of life.

Eccentrics are admired because of their uniqueness and individuality. They are loved by the British and help to make our country so distinctive. They also help to foster respect and tolerance for the differences between people and encourage those who want to express their own eccentricities. The British are fascinated by the quirks and oddities of people's personalities, rather than by perfectionism in humans or society. It certainly makes for a more interesting culture.

Perhaps our acceptance of eccentricity depends on our ability to understand and resonate with eccentric behaviour – there is a line somewhere between eccentricity and behaviour that we cannot understand. Perhaps too a growing public awareness of Asperger syndrome will bring a better understanding of the differences and issues involved, and it will come to be accepted and even admired – just as eccentricity is today.

The extreme male brain

Over the past few decades, society has changed enormously – not least because of the women's movement and the feminizing of politics, business and education, which has led to many changes in perspective on the roles of men and women in society. As we have seen, the prevalence of Asperger syndrome 'appears' to have increased, but are there really more people (mainly men) suffering with a relatively recently discovered disorder, or is the apparent increase due to the changing perspectives of society? These changing perspectives offer several strong arguments for considering Asperger syndrome as simply a difference.

As I mentioned earlier, Professor Simon Baron-Cohen has developed a theory of autism as an extreme of the normal male brain – an idea first suggested by Hans Asperger in 1944. The male brain is naturally better at systemizing, while the female brain is naturally better at empathizing – although we all have both skills to varying degrees. Several researchers since Hans Asperger have also suggested that autism is an extreme variant of the male brain type.

We saw in Chapter 2 how empathizing allows someone to predict the behaviour of another person and to care about how others feel. Empathizing is very subjective, but it is the most powerful way we have of understanding and predicting the social world. Generally, females are much better at empathizing than males and have developed an empathizing female brain type.

Systemizing in contrast involves analysing systems, studying the underlying rules that govern the behaviour of a system, constructing and controlling systems and predicting the behaviour of a system. It requires huge attention to detail. In his paper, 'The extreme male brain theory of autism' (2002),[5] Professor Baron-Cohen demonstrates that there are at least six kinds of system that the human brain can analyse or construct:

1 technical systems: a computer, a musical instrument, a hammer, etc.;
2 natural systems: the tide, a weather front, a plant, etc.;
3 abstract systems: mathematics, a computer program, syntax, etc.;
4 social systems: a political election, a legal system, business systems, etc.;
5 organizable systems: a taxonomy, a collection, a library, etc.;
6 motoric systems: a sports technique, a performance, a technique for playing a musical enjoyment, etc.

When someone systemizes, they watch what happens each time an event occurs, gathering information and analysing similarities and differences between events as well as noticing the outcome. They may conclude that there is a reliable pattern in the system that generates predictable results and allows the formation of a rule about how the system works. If there is an exception, the rule is refined. Systems basically involve monitoring three things in order: input – operation – output. Systemizing is a powerful way of understanding and predicting the inanimate universe.

However, systemizing is practically useless when it comes to predicting a person's behaviour; this requires empathy – a completely different kind of process (and one in which females excel). As a result we get whole books devoted to the subject of male and female differences, such as Allan and Barbara Pease's book, *Why Men Don't Listen and Women Can't Read Maps*, or John Gray's book, *Men are from Mars, Women are from Venus*. It is generally accepted that there are differences between males and females with regard to their thought processes and behaviour. Professor Baron-Cohen suggests that in autism the brain is excessively male-dominated.

In his 2002 paper, Professor Baron-Cohen discusses the evidence for the differences between the female and male brain, as follows:

Empathizing female brain

Females show superior skills in the following, and score higher on tests that measure empathy:

- *Sharing and turn taking*: girls tend to show more concern for fairness and taking turns with others than boys.
- *Rough-and-tumble play*: girls display less rough play, such as wrestling and mock fighting, than boys. Girls show more empathizing in their play, for instance caring for dolls as if they were babies.
- *Responding to distress in others*: females from one year of age show more sympathy for others, while women share the emotional distress of their friends and show more comforting behaviour than men.
- *Using a theory of mind*: by three years of age females have greater skills at inferring what other people might be thinking or intending.
- *Decoding non-verbal communication*: women are better at picking up on body language, tone of voice or facial expressions, as well as judging a person's character.
- *Valuing relationships*: women value reciprocal, intimate and altruistic relationships, while men value status, power and competition.
- *Aggression*: females show less direct aggression than males. In other words females tend to show aggression via gossip, exclusion or bitchy remarks, while men show aggression through physical violence such as punching and hitting (men are also 30–40 times more likely to murder than women).
- *Dominance*: women tend to treat others as equals and share

responsibilities for leadership; men are more likely to establish dominance over others, to push others around or become a leader.

- *Sensitivity in communication*: females are more likely than males to be sensitive, cooperative and collaborative rather than assertive in their style of communication and spend more time negotiating and taking the other person's wishes into account.
- *Talking about emotions*: while men tend to be object or activity focused in their conversations, women talk more about feelings.

Systemizing male brain

Males tend to perform better in systemizing tests than females, and excel in the following areas involved with systems – these include games such as chess and football (body language and conversations are not systems):

- *Preference for toys*: boys are more interested in toys that can be systemized, including vehicles, weapons, building blocks and mechanical toys.
- *Vocational choices*: some occupations are dominated by men, including metalworking, boatbuilding and construction – all involved in constructing systems. Some occupations are dominated by women, such as nursing and primary school teaching, which require a high degree of empathizing skills.
- *Maths, physics and engineering*: these tend to be male dominated and require systemizing skills, rather than empathizing skills.
- *Constructional abilities*: males are generally better at constructing three-dimensional mechanical apparatus and block buildings from two-dimensional blueprints.
- *Attention to relevant detail*: males are better at noticing relevant detail than females, a necessary part of systemizing.
- *Map reading*: males are better than females at reading maps.
- *Motor systems*: males are better than females at throwing or catching moving objects such as balls, or playing darts.

Autism spectrum conditions affect males far more often than females and in Asperger syndrome, the ratio is ten males to every female. This could be because for a male, only a small shift is required from a typical male brain to an extreme male brain, whereas for a female the shift required is much greater. The possible cause of this shift remains unclear, although over-exposure to testosterone during foetal development is a prime candidate and could help explain the theory.

We can begin to see how the characteristics of the extreme male brain may cause difficulties for those with Asperger syndrome. The social world is unpredictable and less controllable than inanimate systems. People with autism and Asperger syndrome tend to react to the unpredictable social world by imposing predictability, trying to control people and systemize social behaviour. This is often the cause of problems in social relationships.

But we might look at the problem from another perspective. Someone with an extreme female brain will be impaired in her systemizing skills. Such a person will have problems in understanding maths, physics or machines as systems and have trouble attending to details – but will be extremely good at empathizing and understanding how other people think and feel. The extreme female brain is not considered a disorder; perhaps with growing understanding and tolerance, the extreme male brain will also be appreciated by society as it once was in our ancestors.

The implied link to Asperger syndrome

As we have seen, the prevalence of Asperger syndrome appears to have increased dramatically since the 1980s and 1990s, with some experts believing it to occur in more than one in 300 of the population. It is found at least ten times more frequently in males than females and there is a strong bias for its traits to be seen in people who follow traditionally male-orientated careers and interests, such as mathematics, engineering, physics and technology. Autistic traits are very common in the general population but only people with large numbers of these traits are diagnosed with Asperger syndrome.

The point is that the prevalence of Asperger syndrome has increased in conjunction with the changing role of women in society and the different expectations we have of men today when compared to our expectations of men throughout history. The traits of Asperger syndrome have probably always been part of the male character, and have been accepted and actively encouraged until recent decades when Western cultural expectations began to change. You could say that Asperger syndrome is a product of our modern age.

Biological differences between men and women

Even the classic, widely accepted and 'normal' differences between men and women can highlight many of the characteristic traits of Asperger syndrome. We all know that men and women are different – not just in their social interactions, but in their biology. This doesn't imply that one is better or worse than the other – we are just different. This is how nature intended us to be. Differences between the male and female brain reflect the biological differences that have evolved between males and females over hundreds of thousands of years. Let's now consider what implications this may have for the condition scientists have identified as Asperger syndrome.

Changing expectations

Human society is ever-changing and developing. In the 1960s, modern women began to want more from their lives and their relationships than being homemakers, mothers and what could be described as little more than chattels to their husbands. Since then, divorce rates have increased, with around 50 per cent of marriages in the Western world now ending in divorce (second marriages are even more likely to fail). Marriage is becoming less and less popular, with the rate of marriage decreasing sharply in recent years. More couples are choosing to cohabit, although many of these relationships are also failing. In the future, it is predicted that more and more people will choose to live alone. It seems that modern humans have very different needs and expectations from those of our ancestors and are finding it difficult to get along. Relationships between men and women are breaking down more frequently in modern society. But how does this relate to our biology and brain structure? And what has it got to do with Asperger syndrome? To answer these questions, we need to look at the differences between the male and female brain and behaviour.

The roles of our human ancestors

Females, throughout evolution, have been responsible for providing parental care to their offspring. The female body was built for child-bearing, and she spent much of her life being pregnant and caring for children. Females therefore are necessarily social and have an enormous capacity for empathy, since they have to understand and predict the needs and behaviour of their offspring, their mate and their social group. Females were also responsible for gathering fruits, nuts and vegetables with other women in the group. They worked as a team and needed to cooperate with each other over issues of childcare and the gathering of food, making good social skills essential. Females had a clear role and were not expected to hunt animals or fight enemies; they were valued for their particular role in society.

Males were responsible for hunting and the protection of the family. The man put himself in danger to provide food for his family and would protect them from predatory animals as well as human enemies. A man's role demanded the systemizing skills of predicting natural systems, such as the movements of wild animals and the weather, as well as technical systems such as how to make tools that could be used to kill prey or build shelters. He also developed the skills to enable him to hit a moving target as he hunted wild animals. A man's role was clear and he was valued for his ability to provide food and protect the family. Nothing more was required of him. He was not involved in childcare or emotional issues and empathy was not necessary. Indeed, it would have distracted him from his role as provider and protector. Empathy can be a hindrance when there are sabre-toothed tigers to deal with!

A typical day for our ancestors would consist of the men going off hunting for meat and the women staying close to the settlement, caring for children and gathering fruits, nuts and vegetables. At the end of the day the men would return with a kill and all the food would be shared. The men would sit around the fire, resting after a day's hunting, while the women would continue to care for the children and keep everyone fed and comfortable. Indeed in some ancient cultures, for example in parts of Africa and Indonesia and among the Inuit of Canada and Greenland, this simple way of life has continued today. Men and women have worked in harmony for thousands of years, and each made an equally vital contribution to the survival of the group. They appreciated each other for their particular skills and abilities and their roles were unequivocal.

Today's society

In today's society, the distinctive roles of men and women have been blurred and we are facing a new order where the rules are still in the process of being thrashed out. Both men and women are confused about what they want their role to be and about what is expected of them. Modern marriage was invented by human society; it is not necessarily compatible with our natural biology. Biologically, a man is programmed to be promiscuous and sire as many offspring as possible with as many different women as possible. A woman is biologically programmed to seek a provider for herself and her children. Both these natural biological roles are in conflict with the expectations of our modern society.

This means that with our increasingly technological culture and shifting social values, the primal skills of males, which were once crucial for providing meat and protection, are no longer required of the average man – we don't need to hunt and kill our own food, nor do we generally require protection from wild animals. Additionally, men are expected to take on roles that were traditionally reserved for females – nurturing, caring for children and being skilled at empathy. They are also expected to be skilled at social interaction and communication, all of which can seem alien to many men and are actually in conflict with their biology.

Mismatch

There is therefore a huge mismatch between our human biology and the cultural expectations of society in the roles of men and women. Like many aspects of our modern biology, our genes have not had time to evolve and adapt to our modern way of living.

Millions of years of evolution developed the brain structures and bodies of men and women in different ways to suit the environment they lived in and their way of life – men as hunters and protectors, and women as gatherers and nurturers. That is our biology. The changing expectations of society, which have distorted these roles, cannot change our basic nature, however much it wants to.

It seems we are struggling to comprehend and cope with the mismatch between our own expectations and ambitions for the way we want our society to develop and the biological reality of who we are. Proponents of the more radical forms of feminism believe that the differences between men and women are purely psychological and culturally constructed. However, science can show experimentally that there are very real differences in brain wiring between men and women. The science and the reality of our biology is not about political or moral equality, nor is it about sexism – either masculism or feminism (masculism is a response by the men's movement to feminism). Science shows that our biology dictates our abilities and skills, and we are stuck with it until our genetic make-up evolves to adapt to our new cultural environment. That could take thousands or even millions of years!

In the meantime we can and must accept our differences and try to understand each other in the best way that we can. It could be that the differences in brain wiring between neurotypical people and those with Asperger syndrome are nothing more than normal biological differences which are recognized and emphasized because of our changing expectations of the roles of men and women in society. Perhaps the people in whom these differences are more extreme are the ones that become labelled with Asperger syndrome.

Some specific differences

So, thanks to the evolutionary requirements I have just outlined, men and women developed differences in brain structure and a different hormonal system, which resulted in a divergence in the way we process information, the way we think, our beliefs, our priorities, perceptions and behaviour. We communicate and interact with each other differently. Biologically men and women are very different and there are hundreds of individual differences – far too many to list here! However, here are a few that are relevant to Asperger syndrome and help to support the idea that rather than a disorder, Asperger syndrome is a variation of normal behaviour, resulting from differences in brain structure and the way that male and female brains process information.

Women's intuition

Between 70 and 80 per cent of our communication is comprised of body language. Vocal sounds make up 20 to 30 per cent, while 7 to 10 per cent is made up of the actual words that are spoken. Women are able to read and analyse body language far more efficiently than men and rely on their intuition and natural skill for empathizing and communicating with others.

Empathy

Women seem to have a huge capacity for empathy – a sixth sense which enables them to pick up on the emotions of other people, even from body language alone. Allan and Barbara Pease, in their book *Why Men Don't Listen and Women Can't Read Maps*, relate an experiment which highlighted women's ability to read body language signals from ten-second film clips of crying babies with the sound turned down, so that the mothers received only visual information. Most mothers rapidly detected a range of emotions from hunger and pain to wind or tiredness, but when the fathers did the same test their success rate was poor – less than 10 per cent of fathers could pick more than two emotions, and many of those were suspected of guessing. Even grandmothers were able to score up to 70 per cent of the mother's score, while many grandfathers could not even identify their own grandchild!

The authors also showed that men and women look for different things when entering a room. In an experiment a number of men and women were each asked to go into a room containing 50 couples. Women were able to analyse the relationship between each couple in less than ten minutes. Women were able to pick up on couples who were getting along with each other, those who'd had an argument, who was making advances on whom, and where the competitive or friendly women were. Men, on the other hand, when entering the room, scanned for exits and entries (a male's evolutionary instinct to search for possible escape routes), the general room layout and items that need fixing or repairing. Women operated on an emotional level, while men operated on a logical, systematic level.

Multitasking

Women are naturally able to multitask. The executive function of a woman's brain allows her to focus on several trains of thought at the same time. A man's brain is compartmentalized and able to focus on only one specific task at a time. This is because, in the male brain, there are fewer nerve fibres in the corpus callosum – the bundle of nerve fibres connecting the left and right hemispheres of the brain. A woman's brain has more connections and allows her to use both sides of the brain simultaneously. In fact many women find it difficult to tell their left from their right because of this enhanced connectivity.

Emotional differences

Allan and Barbara Pease describe how females want relationships, understanding and cooperation, whereas males want power and status and are more interested in things and how they work. In a group of women, you cannot generally identify a leader – they are intent on cooperating with one another and forming relationships. Men in groups, on the other hand, compete with one another for power, status and authority, and there is generally a leader, identifiable from his superior or assertive talk and his body language.

Men tend to define themselves by their work, whereas women tend to define themselves through their relationships and their families. Men are driven to provide for a woman and family, and a measure of a man's success is how much the woman appreciates what he can provide. Women crave love, understanding and conversation and a woman measures the success of a relationship by how fulfilled she is on an emotional level. These differences can cause major problems in a typical relationship, but are accentuated when a man has Asperger syndrome and his female partner does not.

Men and women tend to be interested in different things. Women talk about relationships, personal issues and personalities, while men talk about activities, gadgets, technology, sports and how things work. These differences too are due to the way male and female brains are structured. Sandra Witleson, a Canadian researcher, located the emotional centres of the brain using MRI scans. She found that the emotional centres in a man's brain are located in just two areas of the right hemisphere, allowing him to operate emotional functions separately from other brain functions – a man can have a logical argument without becoming emotional. Witleson found that a woman's emotional centres are located more widely throughout the brain in both right and left hemispheres and are able to operate at the same time as other brain functions. This explains why women become emotional while discussing certain issues. They cannot avoid becoming emotional because of the positioning of their emotional centres throughout the brain.

Emotional upsets

When men become upset or stressed about things, they tend to shut themselves away, either mentally or physically, to try to solve the problem and think things through. This has been described as 'going into their cave' and 'sitting on their rock'. They tend to disengage themselves from conversation and become absorbed in their own interests, whether watching TV, playing sports or pursuing their favourite hobby. This is generally infuriating for women, who prefer to talk about their problems and engage with others on an emotional level. Women feel frustrated and confused when men refuse to talk and retreat into their 'cave', and they feel rejected and unloved when men fail to listen when they need to talk. When a man in a relationship has Asperger syndrome, this trait is particularly accentuated; the woman feels unloved and unwanted, and the man feels frustrated, criticized and nagged.

Men have difficulty coping with women when they are emotional or upset because they feel responsible for finding a solution to the problem, and they feel a failure if they cannot achieve this. Most of the time, all a woman needs when she's upset is for someone to listen to her and comfort her, and this alone will help her to feel better. A man with Asperger syndrome has great difficulty trying to understand other people's feelings and can seem cold and uncaring to a woman who is upset.

The only way to overcome these problems is through understanding how men and women operate under stress and making allowances for each other. Women need to understand that a man needs time to find a solution to his problems on his own. He might shut everyone out and stop talking, or go off and do his own thing.

It is not a personal rejection – just his way of dealing with stress. Men tend to give each other space when they have problems to deal with, but a man needs to understand that when a woman has problems, she needs to talk about it. She won't necessarily need a solution – she just needs talk it through and connect with someone on an emotional level.

Criticism

We all hate to be criticized, but men particularly hate to be criticized because they have evolved to be brave, strong and not show their weaknesses. Man as a hunter had to be successful, or his family would starve – modern men are especially vulnerable to feelings of failure because of this ancient instinct to succeed. A man tends to take even small criticisms to heart and this can explain why men are generally reluctant to show their feelings and tend to bottle up problems. Women, on the other hand, like to help, talk about problems and freely give one another advice as a way to build relationships. Unfortunately, this is in direct conflict to the way a man approaches problems and setbacks, and is the source of much aggravation.

Maxine Aston's research into couples where the man had Asperger syndrome and his partner did not showed that one of the main problems the couple struggled with was that the man was extremely sensitive to disapproval and automatically assumed he was being criticized – even when his partner was simply trying to help. This causes constant misunderstandings between couples.

Speech and communication differences

A man's brain is highly compartmentalized. He tends to store information in a more detached way and has a more logical approach to things; he can easily become confused with the multi-tracking conversations of women. Men look for logical solutions to problems, whereas women like to talk about issues and problems without necessarily needing to find a solution. This causes countless misunderstandings between men and women.

Women also tend to talk indirectly, rather than asking directly for something they want. This helps to build harmony and rapport between women and avoids friction or confrontation – women are able to understand the real meaning of what is being said. However, this indirect way of communicating is widely misunderstood by men – especially men with Asperger syndrome. Someone with Asperger syndrome tends to take things literally, so if a woman is communicating indirectly, or not getting to the point, and a man with Asperger syndrome takes everything she says literally, it is highly unlikely that they will ever understand one another. Women have to learn to say what they mean and be direct in their communication, while men need to clarify what is being said before they make assumptions.

Another source of frustration is that women need to think aloud and use communication naturally as a way to build relationships, whereas men prefer to think silently to themselves and can appear to be distant and uncommunicative. When a man is silent for long periods of time, a woman perceives this as a problem and can feel resentful because she believes she is being ignored. In fact, according to Allan and Barbara Pease, up to 98 per cent of women complain that their men are reluctant to talk.

Research by scientists such as Dr Tonmoy Sharma, a cognitive psychopharmacologist at the Institute of Psychiatry in London, shows that the speech areas in a male's brain are mainly situated in the left hemisphere and are small compared to a female's. A man can struggle with speech and communication because of his brain structure. Women are generally good communicators (both verbal and written) because of the large areas of the brain dedicated to speech and language.

A further area of aggravation between men and women in communication is that women can talk and listen at the same time – in other words, when two women are talking they can both speak and listen to each other simultaneously. They reciprocate and participate in the conversation as a way to build a relationship. Men, however, do not have this multitasking ability and can only talk or listen. They cannot do both simultaneously because of the way their brains are wired. When a woman talks to a man, she naturally wants to participate in the conversation, but a man perceives this as an interruption, and sees her ability to multitrack as being 'scatterbrained'. Men tend to interrupt each other only if they are becoming competitive or aggressive.

These two different approaches to conversation by men and women create huge areas of conflict and can be a real problem when one person has Asperger syndrome, with its extreme male traits. One solution is to make sure that each partner has time to talk without interruption, and that everyone has a chance to talk. Those with Asperger syndrome tend to carry on a long monologue about their own interests, but it is important that a conversation is a two-way process.

Finally, men appear to be insensitive because they do not have the same heightened perception to body language and non-verbal cues that women have evolved, yet the modern woman expects a man to read her body language and verbal signals as another woman would do. Non-verbal communication can cause difficulties not only when Asperger syndrome is present, but when the classic natural differences between typical males and females make themselves evident.

Women are adept at non-verbal communication. They also tend to be very expressive in their body language, gestures and facial expressions; they tend to mirror the emotions of the person they are listening to. Men, however, tend to be expressionless and avoid showing any emotion during conversations, which allows them to feel in control of the situation. They also have a restricted range of listening behaviours. Whereas a woman multitracks conversations, repeating the speaker's words, nodding her head and using a variety of high and low pitched sounds to show she is listening, a man tends to restrict his listening behaviour to the odd grunt. Women accuse men of not listening because they do not give feedback that indicates they are listening – even if they are. In someone with Asperger syndrome, this restricted listening behaviour is even more accentuated.

It's our chemistry

Our biology is controlled not just by our genes, but by our bio-chemistry – a torrent of chemicals that surge through our body and brain from the moment of conception right through to death.

Male or female

Despite the nature versus nurture debate, new research shows that our brain – our basic operating system – is fixed by biochemistry, six to eight weeks following conception, and that our upbringing, our nurture, is secondary to this in governing the way we turn out as adults.

There is a continuum for brain structure ranging from extreme masculinity to extreme femininity, which results in varying degrees of masculine or feminine thinking processes and behaviour. If a male foetus receives enough testosterone to produce male genitals but does not receive enough to fully organize the brain as a male, he will grow up to have varying degrees of the female-type brain, with a more feminine style of thinking and behaving. It is estimated that 80 to 85 per cent of men have masculine brains and 15 to 20 per cent have feminized brains.

The biochemistry of emotions

Some 60 different neuropeptides (strings of amino acids) in our bodies have been found to trigger all our emotional reactions – anger, grief, joy, elation and love are all governed by biochemistry. Even falling in love can be attributed to chemical reactions in the brain that result in the special feeling of being in love. The main chemical responsible for this feeling is phenylethylamine (PEA), which is related to amphetamines. PEA makes your heart race, your stomach do somersaults and is responsible for that head-spinning feeling of elation when you fall in love.

Male and female hormones also affect our emotions and are designed for survival. Men lack progesterone, the hormone that helps prepare the body for pregnancy and childbirth, and do not show the same nurturing response to babies as women do. Typical men can learn to make appropriate responses because they can empathize with their female partner, but men with Asperger syndrome lack this ability to empathize and can seem uncaring and distant.

Men are naturally more aggressive and dominant than women, and this is largely due to their biochemistry as well as their brain structure. If Asperger syndrome is due to an 'extreme male brain', it explains why researchers such as Tony Attwood and Maxine Aston found that people with Asperger syndrome could be arrogant, abusive and had a tendency to suffer angry meltdowns at times.

People with Asperger syndrome can also be exceptionally high achievers and show remarkable focus in their endeavours. Perhaps this is due to higher levels of testosterone.

Adapting takes time

It takes millions of years for genetic changes to take place in a population. The human brain has remained the same in terms of size and function for the last 50,000 years – a minuscule period in evolutionary terms – yet in just a few decades we have expected men and women to make changes to their behaviour which require major changes to the structure and function of large areas of the brain. This is impossible!

Men evolved particular abilities, such as navigational skills and the ability to focus exclusively on their prey without distractions. They did not particularly need conversational skills, social finesse or empathy; therefore their brains did not develop ability in these areas. Women are naturally more adept at empathy and communication. The normal biology of the male brain limits these abilities.

So, despite our changing society and the feminizing of politics, business and education with more feminine value systems, men naturally continue to follow traditional male interests and careers, while women continue to follow feminine pursuits and are more interested in social interaction and communication than men. We are still tied irrevocably to our biology. We have to accept this and make allowances for our biological differences, especially in relation to Asperger syndrome.

Over the last few decades, society has encouraged sexual equality and expected men to develop their feminine, caring and empathetic side – and it is absolutely right that men and women should have equal opportunities in life and be properly respected and appreciated. However, in all this emancipation, has society devalued masculinity and forgotten the benefits that come with a logical, systemizing brain? To redress the balance, we need to find a renewed appreciation of the natural differences between males and females – we *are* biologically different, and that includes our brain and thinking processes. These differences could account for the emergence of 'disorders' such as Asperger syndrome.

5

How to succeed with
social relationships

In earlier chapters, we discussed some of the difficulties experienced by people with Asperger syndrome in social interactions. At a fundamental level these difficulties are associated with the skills and knowledge involved in recognizing and responding to emotional states in others. However, there are a number of positive steps that anyone can take to overcome these difficulties. The fundamental areas that need to be developed include emotions, conversation, eye contact and touch. All of these topics are discussed below.

Reading emotions

Emotions are fundamentally important because they drive and motivate us to behave in a particular way. They have been a critical mechanism for the success of humankind and our evolution into the most sophisticated life form on our planet. Being skilled at reading someone's emotions is highly valuable in social situations. There are a number of tools that can help in building these skills, and some of these are available online and in CD format (see <www.emotiontrainer.co.uk>). Professor Simon Baron-Cohen and his colleagues at Cambridge University have developed an interactive DVD called *Mind Reading: The Interactive Guide to Emotions*, which is an electronic encyclopedia of 412 human emotions designed to help both children and adults with Asperger syndrome to learn how to interpret the thoughts and feelings of other people. It demonstrates facial expressions, body language and speech associated with various emotions. Details of how to obtain this DVD are listed in the Useful addresses section at the back of the book. In essence there are five core skills that are useful to develop:

- the ability to recognize and label your own feelings and know what they mean;
- the ability to characterize someone's emotional state from visual clues and tone of voice;
- the ability to ask someone what they are feeling;
- the ability to assess the words that are spoken in the context of how the person is feeling;
- the ability to decide how best to respond in a constructive way.

There are a variety of emotions that most people experience. The intensity and duration of the emotional experience will vary between people and according to the different situations that they encounter. The outward expression of these feelings will also vary greatly. Some individuals rely on verbal descriptions of their feelings, whereas others give lots of visual clues; body language in general is a clue to our subconscious feelings.

To be successful at reading emotions takes lots of practice and is easier when you can use a friend to learn from. The first place to start is to learn about your own emotions. Study the list below and see how many of these feelings are familiar to you. Can you remember when you last felt these emotions and what were you doing at the time?

angry	irritated	guilty	blue
mad	tense	ashamed	depressed
cross	frustrated	sad	numb
distressed	resentful	enthusiastic	superior
anxious	joyful	peaceful	powerful
terrified	happy	sublime	cautious
afraid	passionate	jealous	contented
sorry	loving	envious	mischievous
hurt	full of hate	perplexed	awkward
upset	excited	puzzled	

Ultimately, it is useful to develop the capacity to know and understand what someone else is feeling, or the ability to put yourself in someone else's shoes. As we saw in Chapter 2, this is known as empathy, and it involves understanding the emotional states of another person on a personal level – not simply recognizing that such emotional states exist. We looked there at the example of having a friend who is grieving over the death of a loved pet, and saw how empathy would involve you imagining how that person feels and almost being able to feel it yourself. If you did not feel empathy, then you might recognize that the other person felt grief, and have sympathy for her, but not be able to imagine how her grief might feel. You could not put yourself in the other person's shoes and imagine being him or her.

Achieving balanced conversations

When two people have a conversation, it will usually have a natural start and finish. When both people take care to manage the 'balance' of the conversation it is more likely that they will establish respect for each other and will be happy to talk to each other on another occasion. The term 'balance' is used to highlight the importance of meeting the needs of both individuals. Several factors are involved in achieving this balance, and they include:

- that neither party is feeling bored or uninterested in the topic. This requires skills in recognizing key body language or verbal clues;
- that both people believe they are being listened to and understood. This is reinforced when the listener paraphrases a message that the speaker is trying to make or asks an incisive question to help expand the understanding;
- that both people are satisfied that they have a fair share of the time to talk and ask questions. This happens when each person recognizes that the other has been quiet and one invites the other to talk about a different topic (often triggered by a question);
- that each person is clearly exploring the subject matter in order to find common ground with the other person.

The other important skill in holding a conversation is to introduce a new subject in a broad sense. It is equally important that you bring the subject to life by referring to the emotions that you associate with it. So rather than starting off with a precise and detailed account, try to solicit some questions so that you can share aspects that the other person is interested in. Why not ask the other person if he or she would find the topic boring before you go too far? Conversations can be confusing and also intimidating and frightening for someone with Asperger syndrome.

> *Jeremy talks about dealing with strangers*
>
> 'When a stranger talks to me unexpectedly, I feel really anxious, almost like I'm under attack. I don't know what to say and I doubt that he is interested in what I have to say anyway. I find it especially difficult to remember names even if I've just been told. When I'm on the spot like this, it feels progressively worse with time. However, what I have learnt to do is to prepare in advance for a series of different situations that I am likely to meet ...
>
> 'First of all, I find it helps if I am gentle with myself and talk to myself in an understanding way. So I avoid in my mind any critical comments and statements like "You must say something back to him" or "I must remember his name" or "I should not tell him I have Asperger syndrome." So if I am successful in being kind to myself then generally I feel more at ease.
>
> 'Another approach that works well for me is to be open and honest. This will take the pressure away because you don't have to keep up a pretence at the same time as thinking up things to say. I will often say, "I'm sorry, my mind was occupied when you gave me your name. Could you repeat it, please?" Alternatively, I might tell them I was "miles away" and need a minute to think about what they have said. It's surprising how understanding people will be and they can usually relate to your difficulties and probably appreciate your honesty. With practice, I have found I actually enjoy talking to strangers on some occasions.'

Eye contact during conversations

Eye contact is important in conversations, helping to acknowledge the speaker and reassure her that you are listening to her as well as expressing your emotions. People with Asperger syndrome can have difficulty using and interpreting eye contact and this can cause misunderstandings. Most tend to avoid eye contact and can come across as uninterested or arrogant.

The website Wrong Planet has some helpful advice on using eye contact, including using soft focusing techniques and making sure you look at a person who is speaking to you, especially at the beginning of a conversation. It is also important to avoid staring and using too much eye contact as this can be interpreted as aggressive.

A good idea is to enlist the help of a friend to practise eye contact during conversations. Ask him or her to be completely honest with you and work together to get the balance right.

Social touching

Touching someone during a conversation can convey empathy. For example, if someone is relating a sad experience and becomes troubled or upset, it can be natural for the listener to touch the speaker lightly on the arm, or even hold his or her hand as a form of reassurance and to convey sympathy. It is more natural for women to do this with each other, even if they are strangers.

However, if you have difficulty reading another person's emotions, it can be hard to strike the right balance when it comes to social touching. People vary a great deal in their preferences for touching during social exchanges. Some people like to be touched, while others feel uncomfortable about touching. If you are unsure, it is wise to avoid touching someone you are not emotionally close to.

If you are upset yourself and need someone to comfort you or support you by touching or holding you, you can always say, 'I need a hug!' Most people will respond to this and be very happy to provide reassurance.

6

Asperger in love: finding and maintaining an intimate relationship

Although it is commonly believed that having Asperger syndrome is incompatible with intimate relationships, people with Asperger syndrome can and do have successful relationships, partnerships and marriages.

People with Asperger syndrome are perfectly capable of love. They have feelings and needs the same as anybody else – they just have difficulty with empathy and understanding other people's feelings, which puts them at a disadvantage.

Finding love

Meeting compatible people and dating successfully is a minefield for most people, whether or not they have Asperger syndrome. For someone with Asperger syndrome the normal difficulties are compounded by the fact that social contact is so much more awkward and bewildering. I'm not sure that anyone finds meeting new people and dating easy – but when you stop worrying about the outcome and decide to enjoy the process, come what may, then it becomes a little easier and more enjoyable. Try to relax and not make a big deal out of dating; it is merely a way of deciding whether someone would make a compatible long-term partner. In the end, you will either find each other attractive and compatible, or you won't – it's about biology and is almost impossible to predict! You may date many different people before you find someone who is right for you.

Traditionally, potential partners have met through social events, friends or work, or through hobbies and interests. People still meet this way, but we now have the Internet, which is fast becoming the most popular way to meet new people. For those with Asperger syndrome, the Internet is the perfect route to meeting someone special. There are many websites and online communities for people with Asperger syndrome, and these can lead to online friendships and real social events. There are also many friendship and dating websites which provide a non-threatening way to meet new people.

For someone with Asperger syndrome, meeting someone via the Internet means you can get to know new people without the hindrance of social inadequacies. It takes away the anxiety surrounding social interaction, and allows you to build a relationship at your own pace. It also allows you to disclose information about your Asperger syndrome, if you choose to, in a safe forum. It can be better to forewarn someone about the difficulties they may face – if they are going to have problems with it, it might be better to get things out in the open early on. At some point, if all goes well, you may want to meet up in person ...

Meeting someone you like

When you finally find someone you like, there are a myriad questions that need answers. How do you know if somebody likes you? Does he find you attractive, or is he just being friendly? How do you read the subtle cues of body language? When is it appropriate to ask somebody out on another date? Where do you go on a date? Who pays? What are the social conventions associated with dating? Plenty of neurotypical people find dating extremely daunting and the great thing is, if you are shy or inexperienced at meeting the opposite sex, it can be very endearing – overconfidence can actually be a turnoff!

The best advice is simply to be yourself. You will either click with somebody or you won't, so pretending to be someone you are not, or trying to play a role, serves no real purpose. Somewhere along the line, your true character will emerge and your tactics will be revealed anyway! Most people can spot someone who is not genuine within seconds of meeting them – it is an intuitive ability in neurotypical people – so if you are acting or pretending, you will come across as someone who is not quite trustworthy. That will ruin your chances from the start and spoil what could have become a genuine and honest relationship.

If you have been diagnosed with Asperger syndrome, have diagnosed yourself or are simply aware of the problems you have in social situations, you may already have strategies to help you cope. Draw on these strategies when you are dating, since the usual social conventions still apply. Additionally, you might find the following dating etiquette useful.

First date

Take the trouble to look nice and be on time – being on time is something that can be a problem for people with Asperger syndrome, so some make an extra effort. It's better to meet in a public place on a first date, but for people with Asperger syndrome, somewhere quiet is preferable to a noisy bar or a crowded party, where social interactions are even more confusing. Perhaps a quiet restaurant for lunch, a picnic in the park, a walk along the beach or a visit to a museum or art gallery would be a good choice. A lunchtime date is a good idea because you can keep it short – your date will understand if you have to get back to work, but will appreciate you taking the time to meet up. This gives you both a chance to see if you are attracted to one another. If you are, you can always make another date.

First date – who pays?

In a modern relationship, it is generally accepted that both parties contribute financially when they are in a position to do so. However, traditionally, the man pays for the first date, and research shows that over 80 per cent of people still think this is appropriate. In evolutionary terms, it symbolizes a man's ability to be a good provider.

Someone with Asperger syndrome may consider this issue purely from a logical perspective and fail to realize how his behaviour is received on an emotional level. A man who wants to make an impression on a woman he is romantically interested in will pay for the first date, without question. When a man expects a woman to pay on a first date, it can be quite off-putting for her and it sends a message that he is not particularly interested in her as a romantic partner. On later dates, you can expect to share the costs more equally.

Make it fun!

Dating should be fun and light-hearted. If you are compatible and a relationship develops into a stronger bond, there will be plenty of time for serious discussions and personal revelations later on. Avoid being arrogant or opinionated, as these are not attractive traits and only serve to make other people feel uncomfortable. Also, avoid discussions on intense or controversial subjects such as religion, money and politics in the early stages of a relationship.

Dating is a way to get to know one another gradually, one date at a time – it is generally considered a mistake to tell your whole life story during the first couple of dates. By disclosing information in small doses, you maintain some of your mystery, and keep your date interested in you.

People with Asperger syndrome have a tendency to hog the conversation with long monologues about their favourite subject without realizing that the listener finds it tedious. Make sure you ask your date questions about himself or herself, and be interested in what he or she has to say. Watch your body language and be careful that you are not sending negative signals, such as eyeing up the waitress instead of your date. Maintain an open posture, use lots of eye contact and smile at your date!

Treat each other with respect

When you meet someone new but you feel that this person is not right for you, treat him or her with respect – enjoy your date and see it as an opportunity for social interaction and the possibility of a new friendship, even if you do not see a romance developing. Consider her feelings and let her down gently if she seems keen on you but you do not wish to take her acquaintance any further. Treat other people as you would like to be treated in a similar situation.

Never pretend to be single when you are not – it is disrespectful and dishonest to date someone when you are already involved in a relationship with someone else. Also, don't discuss past relationships during the first few dates. In fact, even if the relationship develops further, it's a bad idea to dwell on the past and endlessly relive what went wrong. This is true for several reasons. First, if you are still obsessed with a past relationship, you're not over it yet and not truly free to form a new relationship. Second, by reliving all that went wrong in a past relationship, you are simply highlighting your own faults and failings – your date will be viewing things from a different perspective and will see this as a warning. Third, it is disrespectful to your date to talk endlessly about your past relationships – your date's role is not that of a counsellor, enabling you to talk about your own unresolved relationship issues. Consider how you would feel if you liked somebody romantically, but all he ever talked about was a past relationship – it is very hurtful. Concentrate on your date in the here and now and focus on how you can both have fun and enjoy each other's company.

Getting physical

For men and women who are interested in a long-term relationship, it is more respectful – and more attractive – to be rather too reserved when it comes to physical intimacy, than to make inappropriate advances, especially for the first few dates. It is more important for a man to wait for clear signs that a woman is interested in him before he makes any approaches of a sexual nature – and sleeping together before you have achieved emotional intimacy is never a good idea.

However, physical touching is an important part of social interaction and body language and is something that a person with Asperger syndrome can find confusing. Generally, non-sexual touching, such as a brief touch on the forearm to emphasize a point or a guiding hand on the upper part of the back, is an acceptable form of non-verbal communication that shows you are interested in somebody (but make sure you do this in moderation or it becomes irritating!).

A kiss, for somebody you like, at the end of the first date is also an acceptable social convention. It demonstrates your feelings towards the other person and lets the person know that you find him or her attractive. If a kiss is reciprocated, you both know that you feel the same way.

The best advice is to take the physical side of a relationship slowly. A woman will feel more respected and valued for her personality if a man is prepared to wait for sex. And when the majority of men are pushy about wanting sex early in a relationship, a man will seem all the more intriguing and special when he shows he is more interested in getting to know a woman first.

It might be that you have no interest in a sexual relationship. If so you are not alone. A significant number of people with Asperger syndrome describe themselves as 'asexual'.

Martin is content with his non-sexuality

'I feel love, and very strongly. It's just not romantic love. I'm glad that we're starting to realize that a lot of autistic people do want to date and have romantic relationships. I am totally against "desexualizing people with disabilities", but some of us are really not particularly sexual. We can be involved in dating and romance in our own ways without conforming to society's ideas of what is normal.'

Disclosure

Should you bring up the subject of Asperger syndrome? And if so, when? If you have had an official diagnosis of Asperger syndrome from a specialist, you may feel it is better to tell the person you are involved with. We all appreciate honesty and it can be seen as deceptive if you wait too long before disclosing the information. Also, when your new partner is aware of the problems that could arise, he or she is more likely to understand and be prepared to persevere with the relationship. Maxine Aston showed in her research that awareness of Asperger syndrome helped both partners to understand and try to improve the relationship. She also found that if a couple is not aware of Asperger syndrome, or when it is denied or suppressed, relationships are unlikely to survive.

If you suspect that you may have Asperger syndrome but have not had an official diagnosis, it may still be a good idea to discuss the issues and problems you could be faced with, rather than wait until they cause irreparable damage to your relationship. Successful relationships are not easy for people with Asperger syndrome, so it is important to give it the best chance you can. However, it is your choice and you should never do anything you are not entirely comfortable with. Do bear in mind, though, that if you are keeping important information from your partner, this in itself can cause endless difficulties with trust, apart from the added problems that occur because of Asperger syndrome.

A loving relationship

Many people with Asperger syndrome do not form intimate relationships. Not because they do not want them, but because they are fraught with difficulties in communication and social interaction. Even at the best of times, all relationships can be difficult, but when Asperger syndrome is present, the difficulties are hugely exacerbated and it is in the area of intimate personal relationships that most of the problems associated with Asperger syndrome are apparent.

In this section, we will look at some of the relationship issues that can arise for couples where one person has Asperger syndrome and the other is neurotypical, since this seems to be the most common situation. Also, because males are more than ten times more likely to have Asperger syndrome than females, I will focus on relationships where the man has Asperger syndrome and his female partner is neurotypical. Where there is any deviation from this, I will make it clear.

Starting out

People develop loving relationships based on mutual attraction, trust, shared interests and being valued. This is just the same in relationships where one person has Asperger syndrome, but there are some differences and particular problems to be dealt with.

A man with Asperger syndrome is often attracted to a woman based on the fact that she finds him attractive, and this seems to be more important to him than any feelings of sexual attraction he may have towards her. Specialist counsellor and researcher Maxine Aston found that men with Asperger syndrome were more attracted to a woman who clearly showed that she was attracted to him. This came from their need to be liked, approved of and needed – maybe following a lifetime of rejection. She also found that men with Asperger syndrome were attracted to women who were strong, nurturing and showed excellent social abilities.

The progression of a relationship may depend on how well a woman is academically compatible, how she fits into the man's life or whether she takes an interest in his favourite subjects. A man with Asperger syndrome can be very particular about his likes and dislikes in women, particularly about their hair – whether it is long or short, for instance – and his definitions of femininity. He can become quite critical if she falls short of his expectations.

A neurotypical woman may be attracted to a man with Asperger syndrome because he is quiet, gentle, kind and attentive. At the start of a relationship, a man with Asperger syndrome will usually make a huge effort to impress a woman and will go out of his way to make her feel special. Early courtship can be an intense and very enjoyable time.

A developing relationship

Once a relationship is established, a man with Asperger syndrome will stop making an effort and let his true character show. This will result in reactive behaviour in his partner and lead him to wonder why she has started responding to him differently. Both can begin to feel resentful because their relationship has changed.

All relationships change as they develop and the initial feeling of infatuation matures into a more dependable friendship and a more sustainable form of love. In relationships where a man has Asperger syndrome, the change is different – it is more rapid and abrupt because he suddenly stops making an effort. A man with Asperger syndrome may unexpectedly seem indifferent toward his partner and unable to reciprocate on an emotional level. He may become stubborn, seemingly rude and selfish, and expect to be mothered and looked after.

This sudden change happens because a person with Asperger syndrome has difficulty seeing the consequences of his behaviour and is unable to understand how someone else is feeling. He cannot link his behaviour with his partner's emotional reaction due to a deficiency in his theory of mind.

Trust

The question of trust often becomes an issue in a relationship where one partner has Asperger syndrome. According to research by Maxine Aston, 75 per cent of men with Asperger syndrome said they had complete or almost complete trust in their partner, regardless of the length of the relationship, but this trust was not reciprocated. Most men with Asperger syndrome said that their partner did not trust them, particularly in their ability to deal with a crisis, or a particular situation or person. Their partners also stated that they found it difficult to trust them, and found it hard to understand their behaviour because of the ambiguous messages they gave out and the misunderstandings that occurred as a result. Some women whose partners had Asperger syndrome felt that they could not trust their partner or rely on him with issues relating to money, caring for children, being responsible or being safe. This was often because their partner was forgetful, disorganized, or poor at forward planning. However, most women trusted their partners to be faithful.

Despite the high level of trust that men have in their neurotypical partners, many men with Asperger syndrome feel unable to disclose personal information about themselves to their partners. Many say they feel threatened or find it intrusive when their partners ask direct questions about them. Their partners also felt that when they tried to talk about problems they would be accused of being critical. Such problems arise because of a lack of understanding of another person's feelings and perspective among men with Asperger syndrome.

Self-esteem

Most men with Asperger syndrome appear to have low self-esteem and feel that they are not valued by their partners. While they are good at practical tasks which do not require any social interaction or communication, many men with Asperger syndrome evaluate themselves in a relationship and in their social capacity according to what their partners tell them, and they often take such assessments literally, hearing only the negative aspects. They often ignore the context in which comments are made, leading to destructive misunderstandings. Many men say they only feel valued for the logical and practical things they do, and feel unappreciated for the qualities they have, the sacrifices they make for their partners and family, or their contribution to the relationship.

Similarly, most neurotypical women feel that they are only valued for what they do in terms of looking after their partner's needs, rather than for who they are as people. They feel taken for granted, and most feel misunderstood by their partners.

Misunderstandings

Thanks to the tendency of people with Asperger syndrome to take things literally and their lack of ability to see things from someone else's perspective, there can be a great many misunderstandings in an intimate relationship. A person with Asperger syndrome intellectualizes and reasons things out logically, a strategy that does not usually work in situations based on emotions, which are intuitive and spontaneous for a neurotypical person.

People with Asperger syndrome are unable to predict the consequences of their behaviour on their partner and can appear to be selfish, rude and thoughtless – often because they are brutally honest and do not stop to consider someone else's feelings before they answer a question, or make a remark. Where there is a lack of understanding about the issues related to Asperger syndrome, this can cause untold emotional turmoil and confusion for a neurotypical woman and is one of the main reasons why so many relationships fail.

Most men with Asperger syndrome have difficulty hearing and understanding their partner's disclosures about feelings and emotions. They appear to be listening when their partner is describing how she feels, but it becomes apparent that they have not heard, understood or remembered what was said. At the beginning of a relationship, men with Asperger syndrome seem to be able to listen to and understand emotional issues; however, as the relationship progresses, this changes and they become effectively deaf to emotional disclosures. The partners of men with Asperger syndrome feel that they do not understand or care about their thoughts and feelings and eventually stop disclosing them. This can lead to frustration, depression and withdrawal from the relationship.

Most people with Asperger syndrome have above-average intelligence and can learn to say and do the right things through experience and logical deduction, where there is motivation and a commitment to the relationship. Indeed, in a confusing world where people appear to speak a different language – 70 per cent of which is non-verbal body language and subtle signals – most people with Asperger syndrome find it imperative to keep control.

Anger and depression

There appear to be two different types of men with Asperger syndrome: those who become angry and loud when they feel threatened or if they think they are losing control; and those who completely withdraw and become distant or depressed. Both these reactions may be seen as forms of anger and frustration. Depression is anger turned inward in people who are unable to express their anger freely. This coping mechanism can occur in anyone, but appears to be exaggerated in people with Asperger syndrome – their anger either becomes explosive or withdrawal leads to deep depression. Anger in someone with Asperger syndrome can be very unpredictable and irrational and can appear completely out of context.

Explosive anger can be a problem in relationships where one partner has Asperger syndrome. In Aston's research, 70 per cent of men with Asperger syndrome admitted being verbally abusive to their partners, although 40 per cent of these quickly justified their answers with an excuse or reason, such as retaliation to their partner's verbal abuse.

The tendency among people with Asperger syndrome to misinterpret comments as criticism, due to difficulties in communication and understanding social cues, can lead to angry outbursts which are completely unnecessary. Anger seems to be more of a problem where Asperger syndrome is not acknowledged or accepted. Anger is frustrating and damaging for both partners, although it is the most frequent reason given for verbal abuse and can be used as a form of control by the partner with Asperger syndrome. Anger which is passively turned inward can lead to withdrawal, silence and an atmosphere of disapproval which can be equally damaging to the relationship and may cause a build-up of resentment.

A significant number of men with Asperger syndrome have at some time in their relationship been physically abusive towards their partner. These are not extreme attacks and are often carried out in retaliation while restraining an angry partner. Most acts of aggression and physical violence are described as pushing, shoving or restraining, although a few cases involving hitting, punching or kicking have been recorded. Most violence took place only infrequently and it was rare for there to be long-term or chronic violence – it appears to be related to issues of control. In fact most men with Asperger syndrome appear submissive, quiet and non-aggressive, which is what attracted their partners to them initially.

Women ending a relationship with a partner who has Asperger syndrome report that they have felt they were stalked or intimidated by their ex-partner. People with Asperger syndrome find change very difficult to cope with and it is hard for them to let go following a separation or divorce. This difficulty is usually related to issues of control and while they do not intend to be intimidating or manipulating, their behaviour can be perceived as such.

Because there is an expectation in society that women will be empathetic, nurturing and caring, there is extreme pressure on a woman with Asperger syndrome to take on a conventional female role. The high levels of anger and frustration in women with Asperger syndrome may be caused by high levels of stress and anxiety. Many of these women have partners who also have Asperger syndrome, which compounds the problem even further.

Communication in a relationship

Effective communication is vital in any close relationship. But the difficulties that people with Asperger syndrome have make communication, especially non-verbal communication, extremely challenging at times. It is one of the main problem areas in relationships, causing arguments, frustration, misunderstandings and often a gradual deterioration in the relationship.

Some men with Asperger syndrome appear to have very good verbal communication skills, are able to use words in an expressive and articulate way and can be very witty, interesting and entertaining. They can talk impressively about their work or interests and appear to be excellent communicators. However, they tend to see things only from their own perspective and are only good communicators when the subject does not involve interpreting somebody else's feelings, or talking about emotional issues. A man with Asperger syndrome can talk endlessly about his own interests, but will become withdrawn, disinterested or agitated if he has to listen to other people talk about their feelings or about something that is only of interest to them.

It can be difficult for a person with Asperger syndrome to concentrate on anything in which he has little interest. He may constantly interrupt or talk over other people without understanding how rude and unacceptable this behaviour is to them. Hence the focus of most conversations will inevitably turn back to his special interest, leaving the other person feeling deflated and undervalued.

A person with Asperger syndrome may also be afraid to say the wrong thing and can become angry or withdraw if the conversation turns to emotional issues. In a relationship, the partner of a man with Asperger syndrome can end up feeling frustrated, confused and often hurt by these difficulties in communication.

Strategies for communicating

Making a relationship work requires motivation and a commitment by both partners to change the way they communicate and interact. This is often only possible when there is awareness and acceptance of Asperger syndrome. Whenever there are problems with communication, a couple should look at how these relate to Asperger syndrome and find new ways to talk and respond to one another, both verbally and non-verbally.

Adopting a more direct form of communication by being precise and direct about what you are saying can improve things considerably. The partner of someone with Asperger syndrome should learn to say explicitly what she is thinking and the person with Asperger syndrome should learn to read basic verbal and non-verbal signs and not jump to conclusions about what is being communicated. Both partners should have an agreement to explain more carefully what they mean and not to rely on guesswork to decipher what is being communicated. In other words, say what you mean and mean what you say. Avoid ambiguous messages or anything that could have a double meaning or will be difficult to interpret – assume that a person with Asperger syndrome will interpret everything you say literally.

Never make assumptions about what the other person is thinking or feeling. Women particularly rely on their intuition for tuning in to atmospheres and interpreting people's body language, but intuition does not always allow what someone with Asperger syndrome means to be accurately interpreted. For example, it may seem as if someone who avoids eye contact is lying, but for people with Asperger syndrome poor eye contact is common. Those with Asperger syndrome may smile at the wrong time during a conversation, which can seem patronizing, but this may reflect that someone with Asperger syndrome is confused about how to respond. Many non-verbal signals are learnt rather than spontaneous and intuitive and can seem inappropriate when used incorrectly. Where there is any confusion, you should ask the other person to explain more fully what he or she means before making inferences.

Arrange to take turns to have uninterrupted time to talk and listen to each other properly and without distractions. This is important in all relationships, but it is even more vital when one partner has Asperger syndrome because that person will find it difficult to follow several trains of thought at the same time. Try to stick to one subject at a time and avoid a barrage of different questions – take it slowly and cover one question and one subject or issue at a time.

It's a good idea to find time every day or every week to sit down quietly without interruptions from children, television or the telephone to discuss your day or any issues that are problematic or sensitive. Make sure you give your partner plenty of time to talk. It is also important to listen without interrupting or making judgements or assumptions – let your partner know that you are actively listening by repeating back to him or her the essence of what he or she has just said.

It can often help to write things down, either as a letter or an email, especially when there are deep or complex feelings involved. Sometimes it is possible to write about your feelings when you have difficulty expressing yourself verbally, or when there is a risk that what you have to say will be misinterpreted. For everyday communication, a message board can be an effective way to remind each other about things that need to be done, or issues that need to be tackled, without constant verbal reminders that can seem like nagging or criticism.

Counselling for couples

Most neurotypical couples instinctively know and understand each other and are able to empathize with each other on emotional issues. As we have seen, however, empathy is very difficult to achieve when one person has Asperger syndrome. It can feel uncomfortable and unnatural to have to take a logical and impersonal approach as I have just suggested to communicating what may be highly emotional thoughts and feelings. Specialist counselling by someone with knowledge of Asperger syndrome can help.

It is important to find a counsellor who understands and is experienced in dealing with couples where one partner has Asperger syndrome. Counsellors are not psychologists or psychiatrists and are not trained to identify conditions like Asperger syndrome; it is therefore important to find a counsellor who knows how to take the right approach and will have useful advice to offer.

Finding space

People with Asperger syndrome often find socializing demanding and exhausting. Rather than interacting with other people on an intuitive level, the way that neurotypical people enjoy, those with Asperger syndrome need to intellectualize their social interactions and make an effort to learn about and understand social conventions. Putting this knowledge into practice can be extremely tiring, which means that there is a limit to the length of time that someone with Asperger syndrome can comfortably spend socializing.

If you have Asperger syndrome, it is important that you are able to find your own personal comfort zone when it comes to socializing with other people. While it is important to have social contacts and friendships – unless you *really* want to be a recluse – you should not feel obliged to spend too much time engaged in activities you find unpleasant, uncomfortable and exhausting. Everyone can be an extrovert or an introvert, whether or not they have Asperger syndrome, and introverted people benefit from spending time alone to recharge their batteries. There is no reason why you cannot do the same.

Apportioning time appropriately

Many people with Asperger syndrome like to spend time alone, especially when engaged in a special interest. If you live alone, this is generally not a problem – you have plenty of time to do your own thing, with no one else to consider. However, if you have a family or live with a partner, it can cause problems in your relationships when you want to spend too much time in activities that take you away from the people that are close to you. People with Asperger syndrome are notoriously bad at timing, and can easily spend hours or days on their own projects without a thought for anyone else's needs or feelings.

The partners and children of those with Asperger syndrome commonly say that they feel extremely lonely, neglected and unloved when their partner or parent spends too much time engaged in his or her own interests and activities. Somehow, you have to compromise if you want your relationships to be successful. In fact this is true of all relationships, whether or not Asperger syndrome is present.

The best way to please everyone is to negotiate. You need time to spend on your interests, your partner or children need time to spend on their own interests, and you all need to find time to spend together as a family, or a couple.

As a starting point, get everyone to write down their own ideal agenda. It could be presented as a weekly or monthly diary, for example, with time slots for each activity. Fill in time commitments that cannot easily be changed – such as work, homework, voluntary work, caring for a member of the extended family, individual social engagements or regular commitments, important personal chores and activities and so on. Then, around these commitments, try to find periods of time that you could spend together – perhaps through a shared interest, or even attending to regular chores such as shopping, gardening or housework. Actively look for periods of time that you are all prepared to devote to couple time, or family time – it could be a Sunday afternoon, for example, or an evening in the week. Get everyone's agreement that you spend this quality time together without distractions.

Outside these times, it should be agreed that everyone should be able to spend uninterrupted time on their own interests, hobbies and projects. In any relationship, it is important to pursue your own interests. On the other hand, relationships can suffer when too little quality time is spent together – it is all a matter of balance. If you are the person with Asperger syndrome in a relationship, you can deduce this logically. It is not simply a matter of fulfilling the emotional needs of your partner or your children – if you don't spend quality time together, your relationship will wither and die, just as a plant will die without water.

Relating to a partner who has Asperger syndrome

Living with a partner who has Asperger syndrome can be lonely, confusing and frustrating. There may be a profound feeling of sadness that you may never be able to share the sort of emotional closeness and empathy that neurotypical couples take for granted. It can be hard work to ensure that communication is clear and precise so that it does not lead to misunderstandings, especially when social interactions and communication come so easily and intuitively with other neurotypical people.

If you have a partner with Asperger syndrome, it is vital that you find strategies to take care of yourself and your emotional needs. You may have to accept that your relationship will never be able to provide the sort of empathy and understanding that you antici-pated at the beginning of the relationship. Your partner may never be the soul mate you hoped for – that special someone with whom you share your deepest feelings. You may never be able to share your own special interests with your partner, since he is so preoc-cupied with his own, and this can make you feel extremely lonely and undervalued.

Your relationship may eventually break down because of con-tinual difficulties and it is important that you do not stay in a relationship that is destructive to your health, well-being and self-esteem. If you have children, you also have their welfare to consider and it is usually a mistake to stay in a destructive relationship for the sake of the children. There is no obligation for anyone to stay in a relationship that is not working, despite your best efforts – life is too short and too precious for that. In the final analysis, you have to live with the reality of who your partner is, whether he has a 'label' or not. His character, his values and morals, and the way he treats you every day are the things that your partner can make his own decisions about – it has nothing to do with Asperger syndrome.

However, your relationship can be satisfying and fulfilling in many areas, and whether or not it is successful may depend on your expectations. A woman with a partner who has Asperger syndrome is likely to have someone who is faithful, hard-working and honest. Although his need for you will be more practical than emotional, he is likely to be committed to the relationship and loyal to you. If you are committed to making your relationship work, there are a variety of things you can do to make sure your needs are being met.

Maintain your independence

Although modern women are very independent compared to previous generations, some women still become too dependent on a man, not only financially but for their social and emotional needs. This is a mistake in any relationship, but it is especially important to maintain your independence if your partner has Asperger syndrome. It could be a very lonely life if he spends a great deal of time on his special interest, or is unable to deal adequately with emotional issues. Nobody can be expected to fulfil all your needs; it is unrealistic and can be a huge strain on your relationship. So maintain a certain level of independence in all areas of your life. Have your own interests, earn your own money, have your own friends, your own dreams and aspirations in life. Be a whole person, with or without a partner.

Surround yourself with friends

One of the main features of a relationship with someone with Asperger syndrome is the lack of emotional understanding and emotional empathy. As we saw in Chapter 4, for a woman this is a fundamental part of her being. Women need emotional relationships – it is part of their genetic make-up. Men with Asperger syndrome tend to be attracted to women who are exceptionally nurturing and strongly empathetic, so it is especially important for these women to fill their need for emotional fulfilment.

If you have a partner with Asperger syndrome, make sure you maintain your friendships, particularly with other women. Make a special effort to meet them on a regular basis and treasure your friendship with them, no matter how busy life becomes. They are your main antidote to a lack of emotional support from your partner.

Indulge your own interests

If you have a partner with Asperger syndrome, he is likely to spend a great deal of time involved in his own special interest. Even if you both share this special interest and spend quality time together, people with Asperger syndrome can be oppressive and fanatical about their own interests and fail to consider things from your perspective. You may tire of the interest much more quickly than your partner does, and feel the need to balance your life with more varied hobbies and interests.

Try to develop interests of your own. If you have an interest or hobby that your partner does not share, make sure you find enough quality time to pursue it. People with Asperger syndrome can be pushy and controlling about how their partners spend time – make sure you have limits and don't allow yourself to be cajoled into things you're not happy about.

No excuses

Blaming Asperger syndrome for your partner's limitations and inadequacies and the problems with your relationship can be a great coping mechanism. However, it should *not* be used as an excuse for bad behaviour.

People with Asperger syndrome are as capable as anyone else of making decisions about the way they live their life and the way they treat other people. When a problem has been discussed and a clear route towards a solution has been negotiated and agreed, a person with Asperger syndrome can choose to make compromises and change his behaviour or not – the same as anyone else.

People with Asperger syndrome can appear to be very selfish and only consider things from their own perspective – they are only concerned with their own needs and fail to consider the consequences of their comments and actions on other people. This is part of Asperger syndrome and is related to a deficiency in theory of mind. However, there is a danger that *all* selfish, thoughtless behaviour will be blamed on Asperger syndrome with no effort to address the problems it causes in a relationship.

Similarly, Asperger syndrome should not be used as an excuse for unnecessary bursts of anger, domestic violence, verbal aggression, unfaithfulness or blatant disregard of your opinions, thoughts and emotional needs. No one should tolerate continual bad behaviour or stay in a relationship that is making them unhappy, anxious or depressed – for whatever reason. Everyone has a choice about what they will and will not tolerate.

With maturity, time and experience, many of the negative aspects of Asperger syndrome can diminish. Most adults with Asperger syndrome learn strategies that enable them to get along with others, and will come to understand how their behaviour affects other people, their partner in particular – if only through logical deduction and analysis. If people with Asperger syndrome understand how their behaviour affects a partner, and are fully aware of the consequences of their actions, they have a choice about how they behave – the same way everyone else has choices about their behaviour. They can choose to make the necessary effort and take responsibility for their actions, or they can continue to blame Asperger syndrome for everything negative in their character and the circumstances of their life.

Partners and family members can be sucked into a false rationale that Asperger syndrome is to blame for bad behaviour and for everything that goes wrong. However, it is important to remember that if someone is capable of forming an intimate relationship, holding down a career, being a parent or being successful in any other area of life, he is capable of evaluating his behaviour – even if this is done on an intellectual rather than an emotional or intuitive level – and making decisions about how to behave and how to treat other people. Asperger syndrome does not affect a person's morals, his basic character, or his commitment to a relationship.

Mozart and the Whale

The Wrong Planet website recommends a wonderful, inspirational love story called *Mozart and the Whale* by Jerry and Mary Newport, who believe in destiny and in finding your soul mate. A story about two people with Asperger syndrome who fall in love, it details their lives and their love for one another and how they overcame their difficulties and found happiness together. Well worth a read, it was also made into a film in 2005.

Becoming a parent

Parenting can be a difficult time for any couple, but it can be extremely challenging when one partner (statistically, as we have seen, it is usually the male) has Asperger syndrome. Pregnancy, birth and looking after a child can be stressful and unpredictable. There is little room for the rigid routines that give those with Asperger syndrome a certain amount of control over their lives.

Pregnancy and birth

Pregnancy can be an emotionally demanding time, when a woman is bonding with her unborn baby, coping with hormonal fluctuations and her changing body as well as preparing for the enormous changes that parenthood will bring. It can also be a lonely time for a woman whose partner has Asperger syndrome if he is unable to support her emotionally or understand how she feels.

Many fathers-to-be will not want to be at the birth of their child because of the unpredictability of the situation and their uncertainty over the role they are expected to play. This can happen in any relationship, but is accentuated when the father-to-be has Asperger syndrome. This can leave a woman feeling alone and cheated out of a potentially wonderful shared experience, and can add to her stress if she has to worry about her partner when he should be caring for her and their new baby.

One way to reduce anxiety is to include your partner in antenatal care and antenatal classes, and in preparing for the birth. Perhaps he can decorate the nursery and be involved in practical matters such as shopping for equipment and clothes for the new baby. It can also help to write down exactly what is expected of him during pregnancy, labour and delivery as well as in the early days after the baby is born. Clear instructions and guidelines can reduce the anxiety and some of the unpredictability of the situation, and give some control and autonomy to an expectant father with Asperger syndrome.

Baby's arrival

Fathers with Asperger syndrome tend to take on the role of distant observer, with little participation in the care of the baby. Many new mothers prefer to be in control and are happy to become the main decision maker, and do not find this to be a problem. However, other women have reported life after the birth to be extremely lonely and say they have received little or no practical or emotional support from their partner. While this can occur in any relationship, a father with Asperger syndrome may lack empathy towards his partner and fail to appreciate the hard work and emotional demands that a new baby makes. This can cause a huge amount of stress for a woman who feels that she is left to cope with everything on her own, and not surprisingly the relationship can suffer as a result. It is important for a new mother to have emotional and practical support from others if her partner is unable to offer her the help and support she needs.

A father with Asperger syndrome often has problems communicating with his children. He will tend to expect more of them than they are actually able to achieve because of his inability to understand the levels of development and maturity that children reach as they grow. He may have difficulty responding appropriately to children and there may be many misunderstandings and arguments over issues of communication and control, especially during the teenage years, when there can be great deal of disruption in the household as the children assert their independence.

Responsibility

Women whose partners have Asperger syndrome are often left with the main responsibility for the care and upbringing of their children, and may find it extremely stressful when there is so little support from their partner. Many neurotypical mothers feel concerned about their children's welfare when their partners with Asperger syndrome are left in charge of them. This is not because they are worried that the children will be hurt intentionally, but because they feel their partner is unable to be fully responsible for them. Major problems cited by mothers whose partners have Asperger syndrome have included that their partner was likely to become distracted or completely absorbed in something else, to be oblivious to the danger, or not to be able to cope in an emergency. Other problems included not considering a child's feelings and behaving selfishly or thoughtlessly.

A father with Asperger syndrome may also tend to feel rejected when his partner pays more attention to the children than to him. Often, he is operating on the same emotional level as the children, and father and children can end up fighting for the mother's attention. Many mothers end up feeling torn, but a woman's natural instincts will be to defend and care for her children.

Negotiate

To reduce the problems of parenthood, it is important for couples to negotiate rules and responsibilities and set out clear instructions on what is expected from each partner. A large wall chart in a prominent position (such as on the kitchen wall) can be helpful and will reduce ambiguity. List each partner's responsibilities and set out a rota or a diary so that chores are done on time and nothing is missed. Use lists and notices around the house if reminders are necessary. When the rules of the house and each person's responsibilities are negotiated fairly and agreed in advance, stress, resentment and arguments are far less likely.

Communicating with someone who has Asperger syndrome: advice for a partner or friend

The essential thing to remember when communicating with someone who has Asperger syndrome is to avoid ambiguity. It is vital that you are precise, straight to the point and say exactly what you mean. Don't rely on non-verbal cues, as these are unlikely to be perceived – you have to rely on speech or written communication and express yourself in a very direct manner without double meanings, sarcasm or innuendos. People with Asperger syndrome tend to take everything literally, so it is important that you monitor your conversations and check for expressions that could be taken literally and thereby misunderstood.

For neurotypical people, this can be extremely hard work since over 70 per cent of their communication is non-verbal and spontaneous. Their understanding of the various nuances of speech and communication is largely intuitive – they can effectively 'feel' their way through a conversation, interpreting the hidden meanings and the emotional content that is so alien to someone with Asperger syndrome.

People with Asperger syndrome who are able to sustain close relationships are generally highly intelligent and able to develop strategies to cope with and overcome communication difficulties. You can approach problems with being understood in the same way by thinking about them logically. For instance, if your partner has Asperger syndrome and is unable to see how his actions have upset you, you can ask him how he might feel if you did the same thing to him. People with Asperger syndrome have feelings the same as everyone else; their difficulty lies in trying to understand how other people think and feel.

Take an objective approach

Try to intellectualize the problem, rather than approach it in an emotional way – in other words, try to stay as objective as possible. It helps to go for a walk or spend time on your own thinking the problem through before you try to tackle it, as it can be as difficult for a neurotypical person to deal with a problem intellectually as it is for someone with Asperger syndrome to deal with issues on an emotional level.

Make sure you give a complete message, including an objective statement of the facts, your thoughts and opinions about the issue, your feelings about it and what it is you need. Avoid long-winded or rambling speeches. A good way to tackle the problem is to approach it as a bulleted list. It helps to write it down in this way, using it as a summary of what you need to cover. Give your partner a copy of the list when you have finished talking, so there can be no misunderstanding.

As an example, imagine that your partner with Asperger syndrome continually makes rude remarks and is unpleasant to your mother. This is upsetting both you and her. Rather than becoming emotional about the issue, try to remain calm and approach your partner in an objective way, as follows. First, state the facts:

'I've noticed that you frequently make negative comments about my mother.'

Then give your thoughts and opinions:

'I think that this is rude and thoughtless.'

'I understand that you might not be aware of how your comments are being perceived.'
'It is causing problems for all of us and needs to be sorted out.'

Next, explain your feelings:

'I believe that you are not considering my feelings – I feel hurt, angry and frustrated that you cannot do this.'
'I feel that you don't care that you are upsetting my mother.'
'I feel anxious about the rift that this is causing in our family.'

After that, state what you need:

'I need you to realize that this is important to me.'
'I need you to stop making these comments.'
'I need you to make an effort to get along with my mother.'

Finally, suggest possible solutions:

'Consider the nice things you could say to my mother.'
'If you can't think of anything nice to say – don't say anything.'

Obviously, there should be some discussion around these points, and more complex issues will need longer and more detailed explanations. It is always a good idea to write about your problems and your feelings – either as a personal and secret diary to help you cope, or as a means of expressing yourself to another person. A long letter or an email can be a good starting point to address issues in your relationship and express how you feel. However, it is important that you talk things over as well. Just as verbal communication can be misunderstood, so can written material, so it is important to talk to each other and clarify what you mean.

For a neurotypical person, this might seem an alien and unnatural way to approach a problem, but by keeping it simple and logical, you leave no room for ambiguity or misinterpretation. There can be no excuse for your feelings and needs to be misunderstood or neglected when it is approached in this way!

Listening effectively

Avoid making assumptions about how your partner is feeling and give one another time to explain things fully without interruption. Ensure that you take it in turns to speak and that whoever is listening, is listening actively. It can be very hard to listen accurately, and it is a good idea, from time to time, to summarize back to the speaker what is being said. Don't be afraid to take brief notes if you have trouble remembering information and try to respond by encouraging the other person to explain without reacting emotionally. If things get confusing, consider taping or otherwise recording conversations so you can review them together afterwards.

Non-verbal communication

As we have seen, most of our communication is non-verbal, including body language, facial expressions, eye contact and gestures. Neurotypical people instinctively read non-verbal signals and take this ability for granted, but people with Asperger syndrome have great difficulty with this aspect of communication, and frequent misunderstandings and relationship problems occur as a result. They also tend to lack expression and emotion in their communication, which gives a misleading impression and can cause problems in relationships and social interactions, as well as at work. Many people with Asperger syndrome have failed to get jobs that they are well qualified for because of the impression they give at interview.

Crucially, as Maxine Aston's research found, 60 per cent of both men and women with Asperger syndrome were unaware that they had difficulties with non-verbal communication, although their partners reported problems in this area.

It is generally the more subtle non-verbal signals that people with Asperger syndrome have trouble with. The more obvious cues, such as the fact that someone is crying or laughing, as well as clear body language signals and commonly used gestures, are normally read quite easily, while some signals can be learnt on an intellectual level and understood better through experience.

However, for someone with Asperger syndrome, it is impossible to learn the more subtle, intuitive signals. Effective communication can only be achieved by using direct and precise language. This can be a major difficulty in a close relationship, but with acceptance of the situation and practice at the more direct forms of communication, things can improve.

7

Reaching up to your highest aspirations

It has been said that the only success in life is to progressively and consistently achieve goals that are meaningful to you. Success is a very personal matter; it should have little to do with what society perceives success to be – often an image of a wealthy man in a sharp suit and with an executive job in the City. What you decide to do as a vocation in life should be something you feel passionate about, because life is too short for anything less! We all have commitments, duties and obligations to other people in our lives, and we should never neglect these, but with some thought, negotiation and compromise, it is possible to reach up to your highest aspirations and achieve incredible things in your life.

Although people with Asperger syndrome often have narrowly focused interests, they can sometimes make very successful careers from those interests. We looked in Chapter 1 at some examples, such as musician Gary Numan and mathematician Richard Borcherds. It has been suggested that Bill Gates has the traits of Asperger syndrome, and look what a success he has made of his interest in technology!

There are many others with Asperger syndrome who have made an incredible success of their lives by following their special interest – and as we also saw in Chapter 1, there are even more people speculated to have Asperger syndrome who have won Nobel prizes, achieved incredible academic or artistic accomplishments, published books, composed classical music and even changed the course of history. There is no reason why anyone with Asperger syndrome cannot also aspire to reach their full potential in terms of personal achievements and a fulfilling vocation.

You can do it!

In my book, *The Thinking Person's Guide to Happiness* (2007), also published by Sheldon Press, I discussed ways to harness the power of your mind and brain, identify your true desires in life, direct your focus and make necessary changes in order to realize your heartfelt dreams. It showed how anyone can literally 'rewire their brain' for success, and this logical, scientific and systematic approach could appeal to people with Asperger syndrome who are striving to make changes in their lives.

In *The Thinking Person's Guide to Happiness* I also discuss mind blocks, the factors which can prevent us from achieving the success we want. Some of the ways we can deal with these include:

- letting go of past conditioning;
- believing in yourself as a worthwhile human being;
- believing in your ability to achieve success;
- overcoming the fear of failure;
- being prepared to pay the price of success, in terms of the effort involved;
- being objective about other people's opinions;
- developing your own opinions;
- learning to be assertive rather than aggressive or submissive;
- avoiding unrealistic expectations;
- developing the ability to learn from life's lessons and adversity.

Mind blocks apply to anyone who is struggling to achieve success; they are no less powerful for someone with Asperger syndrome. It is worth spending time thinking about your life and planning your future, because each day you spend plodding along and feeling unfulfilled is another day wasted. Take a logical approach to it and learn about the ways you can empower yourself to make changes and reach up to your highest aspirations.

Suitability for employment

As far as careers are concerned, no career is impossible for someone with Asperger syndrome, and many adults with Asperger syndrome have proved themselves to be very capable in mainstream jobs. People with Asperger syndrome have succeeded in careers that range from unskilled work to chief executive posts and have become successful entrepreneurs as well as members of professions including traditional trades, politics, engineering, psychology, teaching and science.

Tony Attwood, in his book *The Complete Guide to Asperger Syndrome*, gives the following list of qualities characteristic of those with Asperger syndrome that make them well qualified for employment:

- reliability;
- persistence;
- perfectionism;
- ability to quickly identify errors;
- technical competence;
- a sense of social justice and integrity;
- likely to question protocols;
- accurate attention to detail;
- capacity for logical thinking;
- conscientiousness;
- knowledgeable;
- originality in problem solving;
- honesty;
- ability to thrive on routine and clear expectations.

Many people with Asperger syndrome have high intelligence and an excellent ability to focus, and can become specialists in their area of work. They make great scientists and engineers and excel in any career where an eye for detail is necessary.

However, while many adults with Asperger syndrome have no trouble getting and keeping a job or building a highly successful career, there are some for whom employment is a source of frustration and persistent barriers, due to the difficulties in social interaction and communication associated with Asperger syndrome. Problems include difficulties with:

- teamwork skills;
- being a line manager;
- conventional methods;

- sensory perception;
- timekeeping and work routines;
- managing and communicating stress and anxiety;
- realistic career expectations;
- matching the job to their qualifications;
- misinterpretation of instructions;
- coping with change;
- accepting advice, which may be perceived as a criticism;
- personal grooming and hygiene;
- fitting in with the group – people with Asperger syndrome may be gullible and vulnerable to being teased and tormented;
- asking for help;
- organizing and planning;
- conflict resolution – people with Asperger syndrome may be liable to blame others;
- interpersonal skills.

If you have experienced these or other problems either while in employment or while trying to find a job, plenty of help is available.

Overcoming barriers to employment

For people with Asperger syndrome who are having difficulties getting and keeping a job, it may be worth a visit to the Disability Employment Adviser (DEA) at the local Job Centre Plus. These officers are knowledgeable about the law regarding disability and can help you access schemes such as the Department of Work and Pensions' Access to Work programme, which aims to help employers meet the additional costs resulting from employing people with disabilities and making adjustments in the workplace.

If you know you are more than capable of doing the job well, yet interviews cause problems in terms of communication misunderstandings, the DEA can also help you to arrange a trial of work instead of a formal interview.

When you are thinking about what type of work you want to do there are many factors to consider. Some of these may not be obvious to you if you have not had much experience of work.

Alison talks about the factors necessary for her ideal work environment
'I have worked as a secretary for a number of years and for different companies. The key things that affect my working environment are:

1   The amount of face-to-face contact with people. I really prefer contact by email.
2   It's best if the office is quiet or else I experience sensory overload. I also prefer natural light and a window rather than artificial light.
3   It's really important that the employer is understanding and accommodating of disabilities.
4   I much prefer managers who can give me written training so I can read it in my own time. It's also better for me if the manager can give me a list of tasks at the start of the week and leave me to it.
5   The staff need to accept that I won't be socializing with them and I prefer it if they don't ask me too many questions. I know that I will tell them about myself when I am ready.
6   I prefer to have my own office, or failing that some kind of screen around my desk.'

Available help for people seeking employment

The Disability Discrimination Act (DDA) 1995 was extended in 2004 to include employers of any size (except the armed forces), which means that all employers have a duty to make reasonable adjustments for people with disabilities.

It may be possible to have a job coach or mentor to discuss problems in the workplace, and the government's Access to Work scheme may be able to provide this. According to figures published by the National Autistic Society, 81 per cent of employers have no understanding of Asperger syndrome; a job coach can help to integrate people with disabilities into their jobs by training work colleagues and managers on the issues surrounding Asperger syndrome, and enabling them to learn to interact and communicate successfully with one another.

These measures have proved to be successful. Statistics from the Prospect of Employment Consultancy (a joint project between the government and the National Autistic Society) show that 67 per cent of their clients have found work, with many others going on to higher education or further training. Most jobs were with large companies in office work and the technical and computer industries. After receiving help to find employment, 98 per cent of clients reported that they were subsequently satisfied with their job.

Case history: Thomas

Thomas Jacobsen was diagnosed with Asperger syndrome in his twenties and works for Specialisterne (<www.specialisterne.com>), a pioneering company in Denmark which is giving people with autism the chance to apply their skills to jobs ranging from IT to product testing. As reported in the *Independent* newspaper, Thomas describes his experience:

> 'Since I started work here, I have learnt to cope better with social interaction and I haven't had a depression in two-and-a-half years. I am getting more involved in bringing new ideas to the company and am part of shaping the Specialisterne Foundation. You do have to have the right environment for people with Asperger's to function – there needs to be an acceptance that I am special, that I might not work regular hours, that I might have down periods – but if you have that in place, we can do any job. Most Specialisterne employees tend to work 20- to 25-hour weeks, but I have brought my hours up to 35. You really blossom here. I see it with so many Aspergerians who join the company and get proper training. I have a lot of friends at the company now, and we socialize and go out together in town. We know we all have that twist.'

Tom's manager, Sonne, talks about opportunities for people with Asperger syndrome in the workplace:

> 'I would be very confident to know there were autistic people running air-traffic control towers. In any company, at least one to five per cent of all tasks would fit well with the skills of people with autism. This could apply to recognition patterns in the medical industry, to accounting, to banks. Of course, some experts have identified autistic traits in people such as Mozart, Da Vinci, Newton, Einstein. If they were alive today, perhaps they would be recognized as having Asperger's, and look at what they achieved.
>
> 'Unfortunately, there is such an emphasis on being a team player and having social skills in the workplace that there is still this resistance. But why do we all have to be like that? There should be room for other kinds of behaviour. My company is

a showcase, but my end game is to get one million specialist people into meaningful work by providing a management model for large corporations to become attractive to people with special needs, so they know that they will be understood and supported. You know, in the UK you spend £12bn a year on the half-a-million Brits with autism. Why not get them earning that for the economy instead?'

8

If you need some help

If you suspect that you could have Asperger syndrome, you may by now have decided whether a professional opinion is necessary or desirable. It is your choice entirely. If you do decide you need a professional opinion, the first port of call should be your GP, who will refer you to the appropriate specialist for assessment.

A number of UK organizations are actively working to support people with Asperger syndrome or autism spectrum disorder. The Autism Trust and the National Autistic Society (see Useful addresses at the back of the book) are two respected organizations that can offer support, advice and help as well as social and employment training and specialist services.

Counselling and therapy

Whether or not you are seeking a diagnosis, you can still get help in the form of specialist counselling. It is important to consult a counsellor who specializes in Asperger syndrome, because he or she will understand what is involved and the best way to tackle any particular issues.

The counselling process

Sometimes all you need is someone to listen while you express your feelings; at other times you may need help with a specific problem – counselling can help you cope and provide a non-threatening environment where you can talk over your difficulties and the issues related to Asperger syndrome. It can help you make sense of past problems and help you to understand your behaviour and emotions in the present. It can also be help with overcoming issues with sensory sensitivity or relationships.

Finding a counsellor

Your GP should be able to find a suitable counsellor; alternatively, there is plenty of help available on the Internet. Try respected organizations such as the National Autistic Society (see Useful addresses section) as the first port of call. They can show you how to find specialist counsellors and set you on the road to getting the help you need. If you need couples counselling, Maxine Aston offers specialist counselling for couples and families affected by Asperger syndrome. She can be found at <www.maxineaston. co.uk>. There is a list of further resources at the end of this book.

Cognitive behavioural therapy

Some counsellors are trained in cognitive behavioural therapy, or CBT. CBT can help people with Asperger syndrome to think in more constructive ways and improve their ability to cope in everyday situations. CBT does not focus on childhood events and experiences, but on what is going on in the present. Because there is not the endless analysis of the past that is characteristic of many traditional forms of therapy, progress is usually relatively fast – often showing results within a matter of weeks. In CBT, negative thoughts and beliefs are challenged, tested and disputed, enabling clients to substitute more positive thoughts and beliefs about themselves and their situation. A programme of CBT typically lasts around eight weeks, and you will be encouraged to make a record of your thoughts, emotions and beliefs in a variety of situations. During sessions with your therapist, you'll be encouraged to challenge these thoughts and beliefs and replace them with positive ones. It is a gradual process of becoming aware of the thought processes that are holding you back or causing difficulties relating to other people.

After several weeks of therapy, you may be asked to practise these new techniques, starting with the easier challenges and working up to situations that you find more difficult. At each stage you will discuss your progress with your therapist, and sometimes with other clients in a CBT group. You will plan each stage carefully and will have control over the way things progress – you will be encouraged to plan your own timetable of change. CBT relies on you to take responsibility for your own behaviour and on your level of motivation to want to change.

Increasing self-esteem

We all suffer problems and bad patches in life; often they are short-lived and we get over them in a reasonable time and return to normal. Sometimes, we suffer a major upheaval or trauma such as the death of a loved one, which can have long-lasting or permanent effects. When someone discovers that he or she has Asperger syndrome, it can be a devastating blow. On the one hand, it can explain many of the difficulties and misunderstandings that have occurred in the past, and in that respect it can be a relief. On the other hand, there is no cure for Asperger syndrome – it is a lifelong condition – and this realization can create a feeling of hopelessness and worthlessness. Self-esteem can be severely dented when someone is diagnosed with Asperger syndrome, but there are ways to improve self-esteem.

Having high self-esteem means that you appreciate yourself and believe that you are worthwhile; it means having a positive attitude, believing in yourself and your abilities, valuing yourself and being in control of your life. Your level of self-esteem can make a critical difference to the way you deal with life's ups and downs and healthy self-esteem can allow you to cope and to get through the bad times.

Your level of self-esteem is a measure of how you judge yourself, and it can suffer badly when you base your opinion of yourself on what other people think of you. All too often, we evaluate and compare ourselves unfavourably to other people. Think about the following questions related to self-esteem:

- Do I like myself?
- Am I proud of who I am?
- Am I proud of what I'm doing with my life?
- Am I a decent human being?
- Do I deserve to be loved?
- Do I deserve to be happy?
- Do I accept my faults and limitations?
- Do I recognize that nobody is perfect – that we all have our faults?
- Do I believe that my opinions are as valid as anybody else's?
- Do I believe I am as good as anybody else?

- Do I treat myself and others with respect?
- Am I committed to self-improvement?
- Do I take responsibility for myself and my actions?

To improve your self-esteem you need to work on positive answers to these questions. Healthy self-esteem depends on self-understanding and self-acceptance. You have to gain perspective and judge your goals and aspirations independently of society and other people at large. Strive to always behave in a way that you can feel proud of – learn to love who you are!

Be true to yourself

To be happy, it is important to be true to yourself and to have goals and plans that you are deeply committed to and passionate about. You have to have something you can believe in and stand up for – you have to find your purpose in life and strive to reach your highest aspirations.

If you are continually fighting with your own personality, worrying about being different and trying constantly to become something or someone that is impossible to achieve, you will be unhappy, frustrated, depressed and unfulfilled. It is vital that you accept who you are and look for the good things about your situation and about your life. We all have flaws in our personality and issues from the past that we struggle to cope with – think of having Asperger syndrome as just another challenge in life.

Discover all the positive things about yourself and learn how to value yourself for who you are. Stop worrying about the labels people put on you. If you continually worry about things you cannot change, you will create barriers to any success in life, in relationships and in work. You can make a valuable contribution to the world just by being yourself. Focus on the positive aspects and think of all the benefits that having Asperger syndrome can have.

Finally ...

Remember, Asperger syndrome has been classified as a disorder or a disability – however, it is only considered a disability because everyone is expected to have the same level of social ability.

As we saw in Chapter 4, the problem is that society has changed, but our biology hasn't. People with Asperger syndrome are expected to fit in with the expectations of our modern society, but they literally have to pretend to be 'normal' – they have to work hard to appear to be the same as the neurotypical population. It is just not possible for anyone to change their brain structure to fit in with the expectations of a changing society!

[Asperger syndrome is not a problem among other people with Asperger syndrome – it is only a problem for people who are classed as neurotypical and are unable to understand how information is processed differently in atypical individuals.] A change of perspective is all that is needed for people to see the many benefits of knowing and loving someone who has Asperger syndrome, rather than dwelling on the problems.]

In our modern technological society, the characteristics of Asperger syndrome, such as attention to detail and systems, are becoming more highly prized, for example in computer sciences. The revolution in computer technology in the twentieth and twenty-first centuries has opened up extraordinary opportunities for people with the specialized skills and attributes characteristic of Asperger syndrome. [A person with Asperger syndrome has many abilities that are indispensable in the modern world, relating to skills that include maths, science, engineering, computing, linguistics and music. In fact, we could speculate that the numbers of people with skills that lead to success in these areas might increase in the future.]

So embrace who you are and reach up to your highest aspirations. Believe in yourself and your abilities. After all, [it is only a matter of opinion as to whether Asperger syndrome is a disorder or simply a natural biological difference]...

References

1 Baron-Cohen, S., Wheelwright, S., Robinson, J. and Woodbury Smith, M. (2005). 'The adult Asperger assessment (AAA): a diagnostic method'. *Journal of Autism and Developmental Disorders* 35, 807–19.
2 <http://www.autism.com/families/therapy/visual.htm>.
3 Baron-Cohen, S., et al. (2005). 'The adult Asperger assessment (AAA)'.
4 <http://www.autism.com/families/therapy/visual.htm>.
5 Baron-Cohen, S. (2002). 'The extreme male brain theory of autism'. *Trends in Cognitive Sciences* 6.6.

Useful addresses

General

The Autism Trust
29A Stafford Street
Edinburgh EH3 7BJ
Tel.: 0131 558 7444
Fax: 0131 476 3170
Email: admin@autismtrust.org.uk
Website: www.autismtrust.org.uk

45 Nightingale Road
Hampton
Middlesex TW12 3HX
Tel.: 020 8783 3714
Email: info@theautismtrust.org.uk
Website: www.theautismtrust.com

National Autistic Society (NAS)
393 City Road
London EC1V 1NG
Tel.: 020 7833 2299
Helpline: 0845 070 4004
Website: www.nas.org.uk

The Autism Services Directory also comes under the auspices of NAS: visit
its own website <www.autismdirectory.org.uk>.

Disability Law Service
39–45 Cavell Street
London E1 2BP
Tel.: 020 7791 9800 (advice line: 10 a.m. to 5 p.m., Monday to Friday)
Website: www.dls.org.uk

Disability Rights Commission *see* **Equality and Human Rights
Commission**

Employers' Forum on Disability
Nutmeg House
60 Gainsford Street
London SE1 2NY
Tel.: 020 7403 3020
Website: www.efd.org.uk

Equality and Human Rights Commission
Arndale House
The Arndale Centre
Manchester M4 3AQ
Tel.: 0161 829 8100
Helpline: 0845 604 6610
Website: www.equalityhumanrights.com

Mind (National Association for Mental Health)
Granta House
15–19 Broadway
Stratford
London E15 4BQ
Tel.: 020 8519 2122
Mind*info*Line: 0845 766 0163
Website: www.mind.org.uk

Mind Reading
An interactive reference work covering the entire spectrum of human emotions, and which is distributed by Jessica Kingsley Publishers.
Website: www.jkp.com/mindreading

Prospects Employment Service
Tel.: 020 7704 7450
Email: prospects:london@nas.org.uk
Further details may be accessed through the National Autistic Society website.

Specialisterne
Website: www.specialisterne.com

A Danish IT company that assesses and trains people with ASD, using their particular skills and characteristics to improve the quality of its software testing.

Counselling – individuals and organizations

Maxine Aston specializes in working with individuals, couples and families with Asperger syndrome, and she also arranges and leads workshops.
Website: www.maxineaston.co.uk

Tony Attwood is a British psychologist and writer living in Queensland. His website <www.tonyattwood.com.au> is a guide for people with Asperger syndrome and their families, and also for professionals.

British Association for Behavioural and Cognitive Psychotherapies
Victoria Buildings
9–13 Silver Street
Bury BL9 0EU
Tel.: 0161 797 4484
Website: www.babcp.com

British Association of Counselling and Psychotherapy
Tel.: 01455 883316
Website: www.bacp.co.uk

British Psychological Society
Tel.: 0116 254 9568
Website: www.bps.org.uk

Chris and Gisela Slater-Walker are a married couple, one of whom has Asperger syndrome. They are the authors of several books on the condition, and they also offer relationship advice.
Website: www.asperger-marriage.info

Further reading

Aston, M., *Aspergers in Love: Couple relationships and family affairs*. London, Jessica Kingsley Publishers, 2003.

Aston, M., *The Other Half of Asperger Syndrome*. London, National Autistic Society, 2001.

Attwood, T., *The Complete Guide to Asperger's Syndrome*. London, Jessica Kingsley Publishers, 2007.

Baron-Cohen, S., 'Is Asperger syndrome necessarily a disability?' Based on an essay first published in *Development and Psychopathology*, 12 (2000), 489–500.

Gray, J., *Men are from Mars, Women are from Venus: A practical guide for improving communication and getting what you want in your relationships*. London, Thorsons Publishers, 1993.

Lawson, W., *Life Behind Glass*. London, Jessica Kingsley Publishers, 1998.

Pease, A. and Pease, B., *Why Men Don't Listen and Women Can't Read Maps: How we're different and what to do about it*. London, Orion, 2001.

Searle, R., *The Thinking Person's Guide to Happiness*. London, Sheldon Press, 2007.

Willey, L. H., *Pretending to be Normal: Living with Asperger's syndrome*. London, Jessica Kingsley Publishers, 1999.

Index